Creating An Inspired Life Through Yoga

YOU DON'T HAVE TO STAND ON YOUR HEAD

By Dee Gold
Photography by Jim Guzel

Inner Reaches Press   •   *North Potomac, MD*   •   *2009*

You Don't Have to Stand on Your Head:

Creating an Inspired Life Through Yoga

Copyright © 2009 by Dee Gold.

Photography copyright © 2009 by Jim Guzel.

Design by Bonotom Studio, Inc.
Arlington, VA 22201

Printed in the United States of America by
Chakra Communications, Buffalo, NY 14203

ISBN 978-0-9821782-1-8

HEA025000

Library of Congress Control Number:
2009932247

THIS BOOK IS DEDICATED TO THE CREATIVE SPIRIT.

Five years in the making, this project has been a labor of love from beginning to end. It was a love of yoga that started it all. It was the love of friends and family that sustained me through the many ups and downs and ins and outs. I owe thanks to so many that it would be impossible to fit them all on one page but there are those whose support and generosity have been remarkably steady and invaluable. They must be mentioned.

Thanks, first to **ALL THE MODELS** who so courageously stripped away their inhibitions to give their all, with little compensation, to a project that sometimes felt as though it would never come to fruition. Your belief in me and your trust in the process got me through.

Thank you, **JIM**, for the gorgeous photos and the great adventure!

Thank you, **ANN** and **DAN**, for weaving your word magic and teaching me the art of conciseness. I love you both!

To **LISA** and **JUSTIN**, thank you for jump-starting the design and for your loving support throughout.

To my dear friends, **COURTNEY** and **CECE**, thank you for being unwavering cheerleaders.

Thank you **PATTY**, for your grace and wisdom and for **BONO**. Thank you Bono, for your generosity, professionalism, and for **ABIGAIL**. Thank you Abigail for your skill and your sunny smile.

Thank you **LEE**, for your loving support and for **CHARLIE**. Thank you Charlie, for your kindness and for **SHARIQUE**. Thank you Sharique, for your graciousness and expertise.

Thank you to my many teachers and guides, including **MARILYN**, **BRUCE**, the folks at **INTEGRAL INSTITUTE** and **PHOENIX RISING YOGA THERAPY**. I bow in gratitude to the great yoga masters and sages throughout history, without whom there would be no foundation for this book.

ABBY, where would I be without you? Thank you for taking over the studio and allowing me to focus on the book.

MOM and **DAD**, thank you for believing in me even when you didn't quite understand me.

LILLIAN, **WARREN**, **STEPHANIE**, and **STEVE**, I miss you and feel inspired by you every day. Thank you for your enduring presence.

To my cherished children, **JOSH** and **KATE**, your abiding faith in me was the ground on which I walked from start to finish. Thank you so much! I adore you both.

Thank you to MY GYM in Gaithersburg, Maryland for the use of your inspiring indoor playground!

And finally, to the archetypal Fool. Thank you for whispering in my ear that I could write a book and for keeping me laughing along the way.

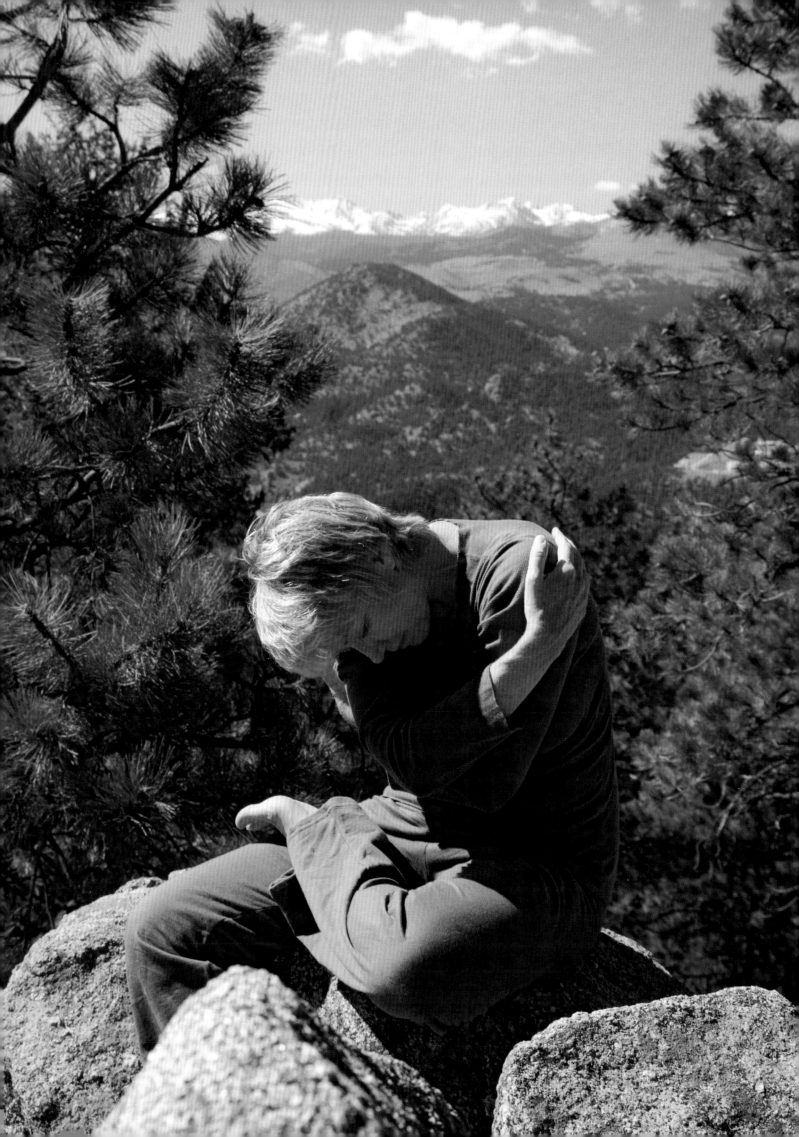

DEE GOLD HAS BEEN
TEACHING HATHA YOGA
FOR MORE THAN 25 YEARS.
Her love of creative movement grew out of
her modern dance training. After studying
psychology in college, she earned a Masters
Degree in dance-movement therapy.

Dee teaches yoga in the Washington,
DC area at her studio, Inner Reaches
Yoga & Health in Gaithersburg,
Maryland. Her yoga retreats and stress
management seminars have become
legendary in the famously workaholic
capital, and her clients include business
executives, journalists, lobbyists, medical
professionals, nonprofit groups, sports
professionals, counselors, educators,
teenagers, parents and the elderly.

You Don't Have To Stand On Your Head
was inspired by Dee's often stressed and
overworked students, who urged her to
share her unique approach by showing
how individuals can joyfully and playfully
explore their minds, bodies and spirits.
She seeks to encourage a creative practice
of yoga that students can easily take into
the world outside the yoga studio.

The mother of two adult children, Dee
lives in North Potomac, Maryland.

Namaste ♡
De Gold
2010

5

ABOUT THE AUTHOR

YOGA
FOR
EVERY
BODY

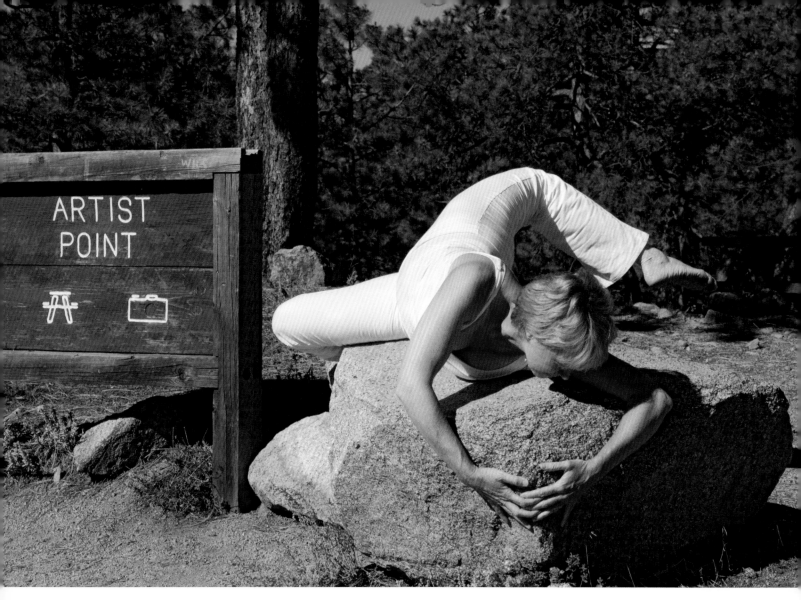

HEAR THE WORD "YOGA" AND WHAT DO YOU PICTURE?

Perhaps stylish young women dressed in lycra, limber as gymnasts, or ultra flexible, muscular young men contorting their bodies or standing on their heads. In fact, as you'll see in this book, yoga is for every body, regardless of age or physical condition (that's me in the photo, age 54)

The models pictured in this book are ordinary people of all ages and levels of fitness with varied interests and busy lives. Their experience with yoga ranges from beginner, to erratic practitioner, to dedicated student, to accomplished teacher. What they have in common is that they have accepted my invitation to stretch beyond the confines of their yoga mats to enrich their lives by artistically creating their own yoga.

The creative art of yoga is the expressive art of the soul. The word "yoga," in Sanskrit means "yoke" or "union" and the formal practice of yoga, with roots in ancient India, is a discipline that unites body and mind as a path toward spiritual enlightenment. Texts translated from the original Sanskrit provide evidence of the practice of yoga dating back more than eight thousand years.

But what gave rise to yoga? I link the formal practice of yoga with a primal human capacity. Picture prehistoric humans exploring their place in the world by "trying on" forms that they saw around them, forms which contained the "spirits" of animals and objects in their environment. By eating the meat of an animal an individual might have hoped to attain its vital qualities. By assuming the shape of an object one might embody its essence. Connected with their environment in this way early humans could acquire the agility of a snake, the stability of a mountain and the stealth of predatory animals. Through repeated practice these attributes could be strengthened, enhancing and empowering human existence.

Some modern Native Americans, like their ancestors, embark on personal vision quests in search of their "power animal" and appeal to the spirit of the animal to inhabit their human form. I see that as an expression of yoga. As a part of their spiritual observance, current-day Ticunas in the Amazon basin enact a trip through the jungle, mimicking the creatures they encounter along the way. Isn't that a form of yoga?

Connecting with nature and "Spirit" seems to be an innate human desire. Witness children of all cultures as they gallop as horses, wriggle as worms and flap their arms to fly as birds. Is there any doubt of the inspired quality of such play? We humans have a natural tendency to engage our imaginations in joyful pursuit of union with the environment as a way to activate our connection to Spirit. This, to me, is pure yoga.

That humans learn by mimicking is well documented. The ability to do so seems to be genetically inherited, suggesting its importance

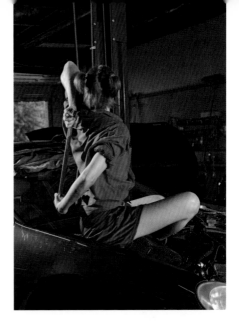

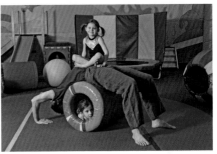

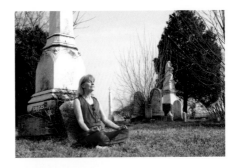

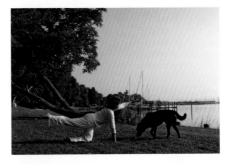

12

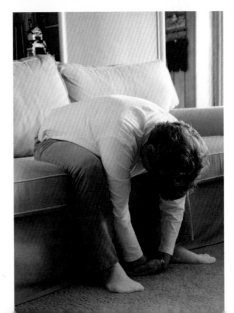

to survival. But something mysterious can happen when body and mind join together in this way, something that eludes language and expands conscious awareness beyond ordinary experience and simple survival concerns. Over the course of human history we've come to describe that mystery as "spiritual experience." As the ancient Hindus realized, the union of body and mind gives rise to conscious awareness of Spirit.

Taoists throughout the ages have engaged in the practice of meditating on nature in order to unite with the Divine. Transcending ordinary human consciousness, they "become" the river, the mountain or the wind. Certain Buddhists seek to empty their minds by sitting in stillness as a way of realizing their divine nature. Like these spiritual seekers, each of us has the capacity to quiet our internal chatter, liberate ourselves from the tyranny of inhibiting self-judgment and experience ourselves as sacred expressions of life. Yoga offers a path toward such liberation.

While the formal practice of yoga typically adheres to strict teachings that stem directly from ancient Hindu philosophy, nothing should stand in the way of you and I artistically creating a personal practice inspired by the purest meaning of the word "yoga." In essence, a creative practice of uniting mind and body in service of spiritual experience might closely resemble the primitive practice of mimicking movement and shapes found in our surroundings to embody the power of Spirit.

In contemporary Western culture we may have temporarily lost touch with our innate ability to unite with the Divine in this way. With our concern for physical fitness many have appropriately turned to yoga as a tool for losing weight, increasing strength and improving flexibility. Western medicine has embraced yoga as an effective method for health management with proven benefits for patients suffering high blood pressure, arthritis, chronic pain, mood disorders, ulcers and a variety of other ailments. Yoga, from this perspective, can be seen as an important survival tool. But, to me, the most exciting aspect of yoga is that it can take the practitioner beyond survival, beyond fitness and wellness, into the realm of spiritual mystery and wonder.

Without losing sight of the many documented health benefits and without minimizing the reverence of ancient spiritual practices and the attainments of beloved yoga masters, witness in the coming pages the

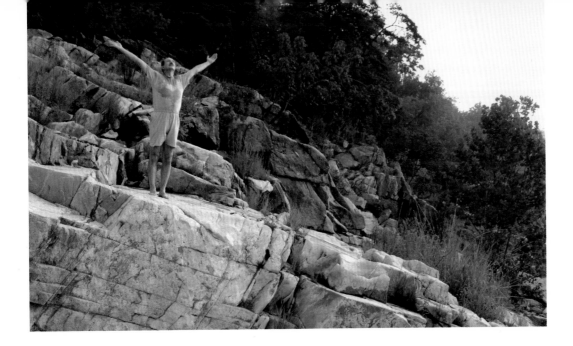

power of a personal practice taken off the traditional yoga mat which unites mind and body in spontaneous play with Spirit.

My philosophy, as a yoga student, practitioner and teacher, is that life is a blank canvas for the soul. Each soul has a sacred drive to create. Each human consciousness contains within it the artistry needed to successfully complete a masterpiece. While yoga embodies direct knowledge of form, shape and context the masterpiece is created when mind and body unite with Spirit. In other words, yoga inspires a masterful life enriched through exploration, experimentation and play.

Through this type of exploration yoga can be a way to connect with kindred spirits or to deepen into a more loving relationship with another. Yoga means union. You can adapt it to summon the forces of nature, embracing the sun's warmth or receiving the spray of the sea. You can dance your yoga, become one with a sailboat, bring richness to daily chores or realize your tree-goddess nature. Horse around in a field of buttercups or monkey around with wrenches. Become the key to unlock the beauty of life or come to grips with the transition we call death. Yoga, when practiced in this way, is an artistic expression of the individual soul in union with the Divine.

I hope this book will inspire every reader to practice yoga. If you already have a practice, no matter how advanced, I hope you'll stretch beyond your mat to playfully explore your creative spirit. If you've never practiced but feel inspired by what you see here I encourage you to seek out a teacher who can acquaint you with the fundamentals of a traditional yoga practice, establishing a safe and sound foundation from which to spring.

Please accept my invitation to playfully transcend all preconceived notions about yoga. Like the individuals you are about to meet in the coming pages you can artistically bring your yoga to life and enhance your day-to-day existence simply by opening to the possibility of engaging Spirit through creative interaction with your environment.

Yoga, like life, is a never-ending emergence. Reach beyond the confines of the ordinary and participate in Divine creation. Discover the artistic nature of your body, mind and spirit. Explore. Engage. Express! Above all, remember that you are the artist. Yoga is the art.

You don't have to stand on your head ... but you can if you're inspired to!

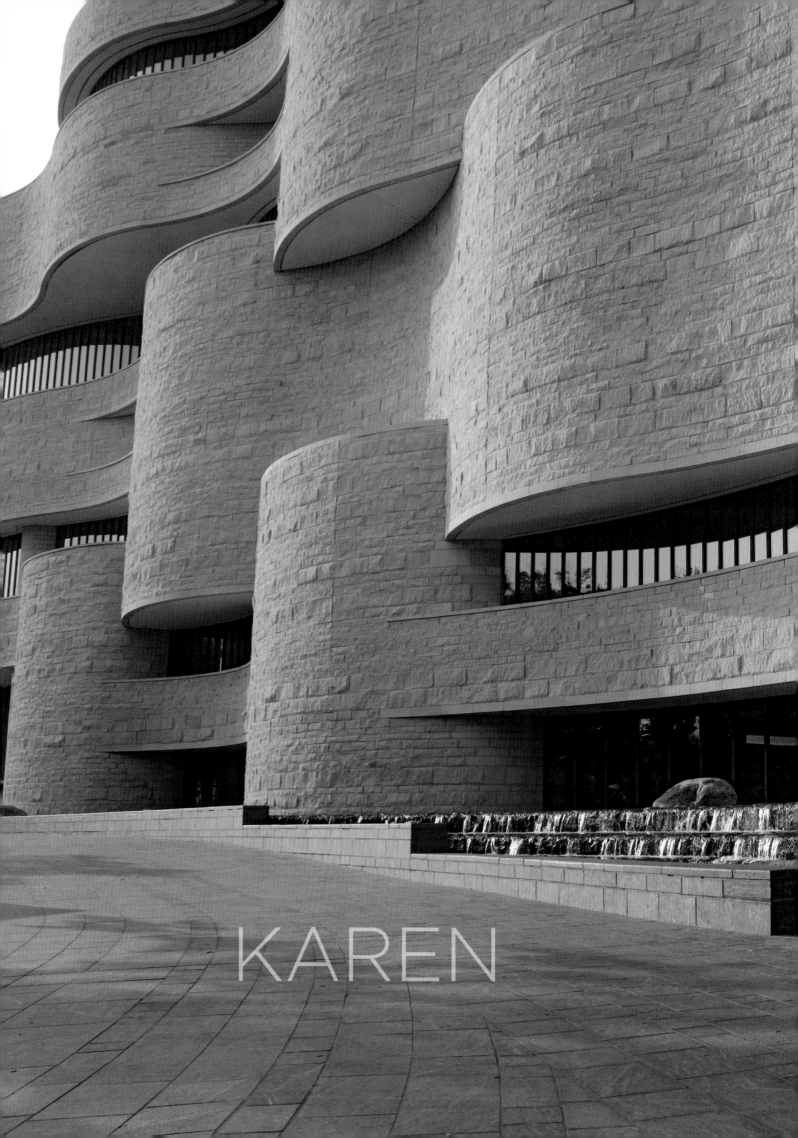

KAREN

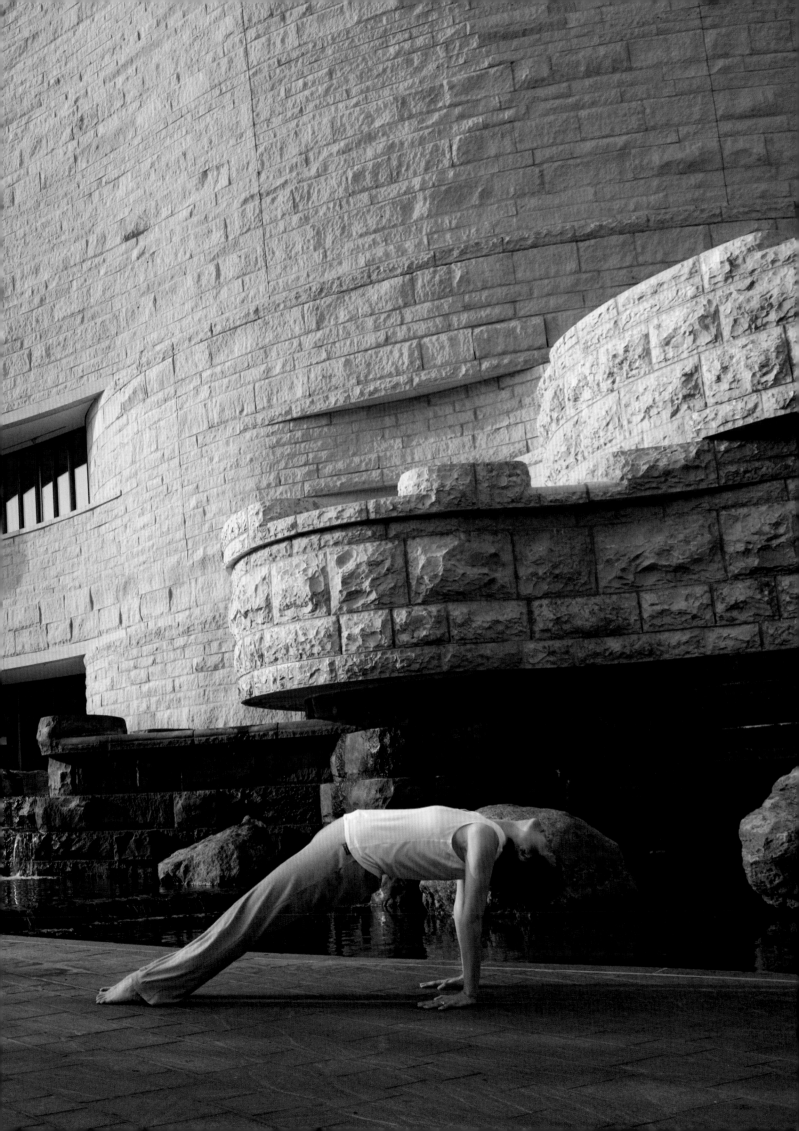

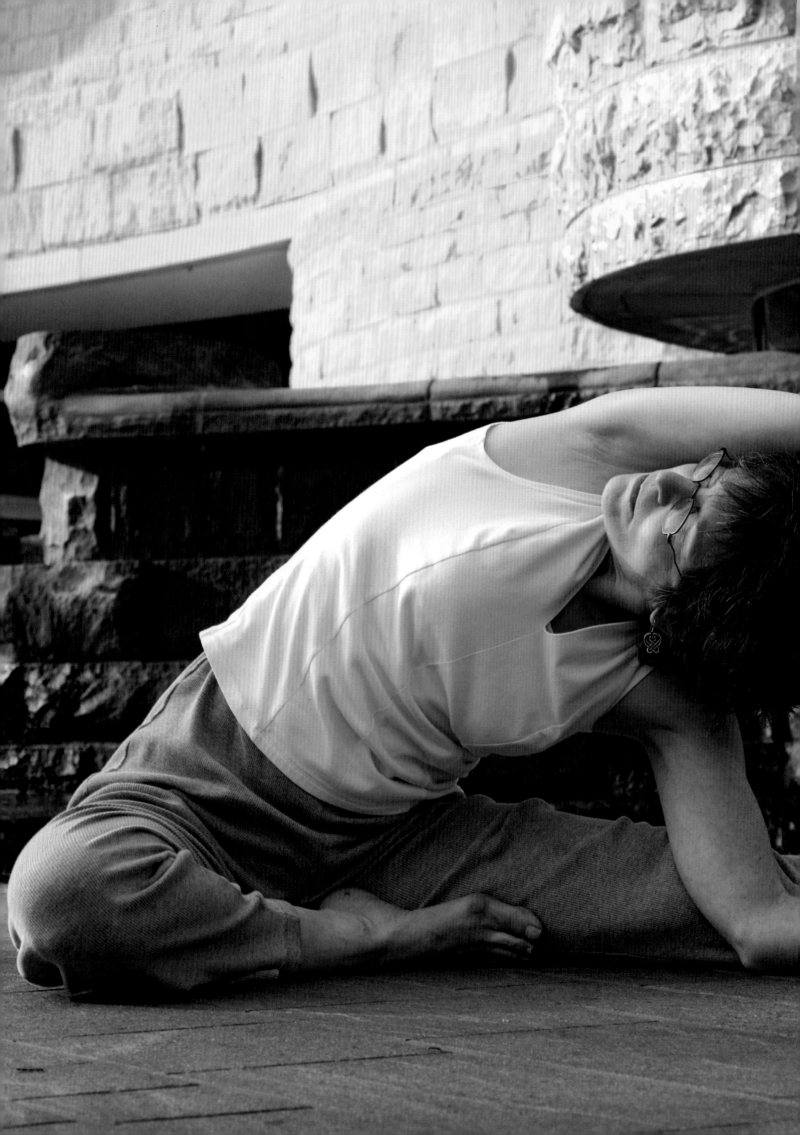

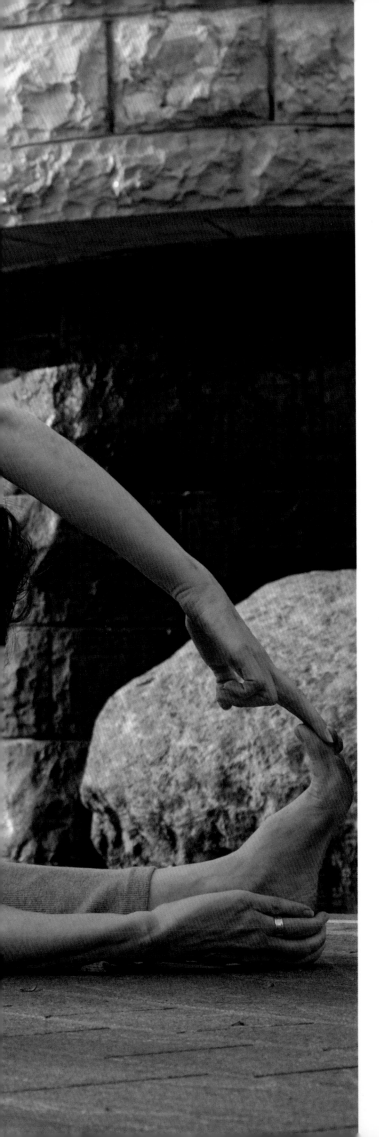

WHEN KAREN WAS INVITED TO TAKE HER YOGA "OFF THE MAT"

she responded with characteristic enthusiasm. This high-energy, 53-year-old executive coach delights in freedom of expression. "Yoga off the mat?" she thought. "This could be fun!" Embracing the challenge, she chose to practice her yoga on the grounds of the Smithsonian Institution in Washington, D.C., identifying it as "a peaceful retreat amid the hustle and bustle of a busy, urban life."

At 45, Karen turned to yoga hoping to learn to relax both body and mind. Her aerobic exercise routine had kept her heart healthy and helped her cope with stress. But the muscles of her legs and lower back had become so tight that her reach barely extended below her knees in a forward bend. The hunch of her shoulders caused her chest to cave slightly, creating a "C" curve in her upper back. Her massage therapist suggested she try yoga.

"Before yoga," she says, "I never stopped. My mind was always focused on the next thing." She says that yoga has helped her develop the patience to be still. "I've discovered that stillness is liberating. The stillness of a yoga pose can quiet the mind. A quiet mind can be a conduit for creative self-expression."

Karen found inspiration in the shapes and textures surrounding her at the Smithsonian. The Moon Gate outside the Sackler Museum was especially intriguing. "This hard granite structure had movement," she says. "It was amazing! I sensed a gentle vibration pulsating, as if the shape of the circle created a powerful energy flow. It was exactly like a yoga pose. When I'm in the stillness of a pose I feel a subtle energy running through me and I am set free."

17

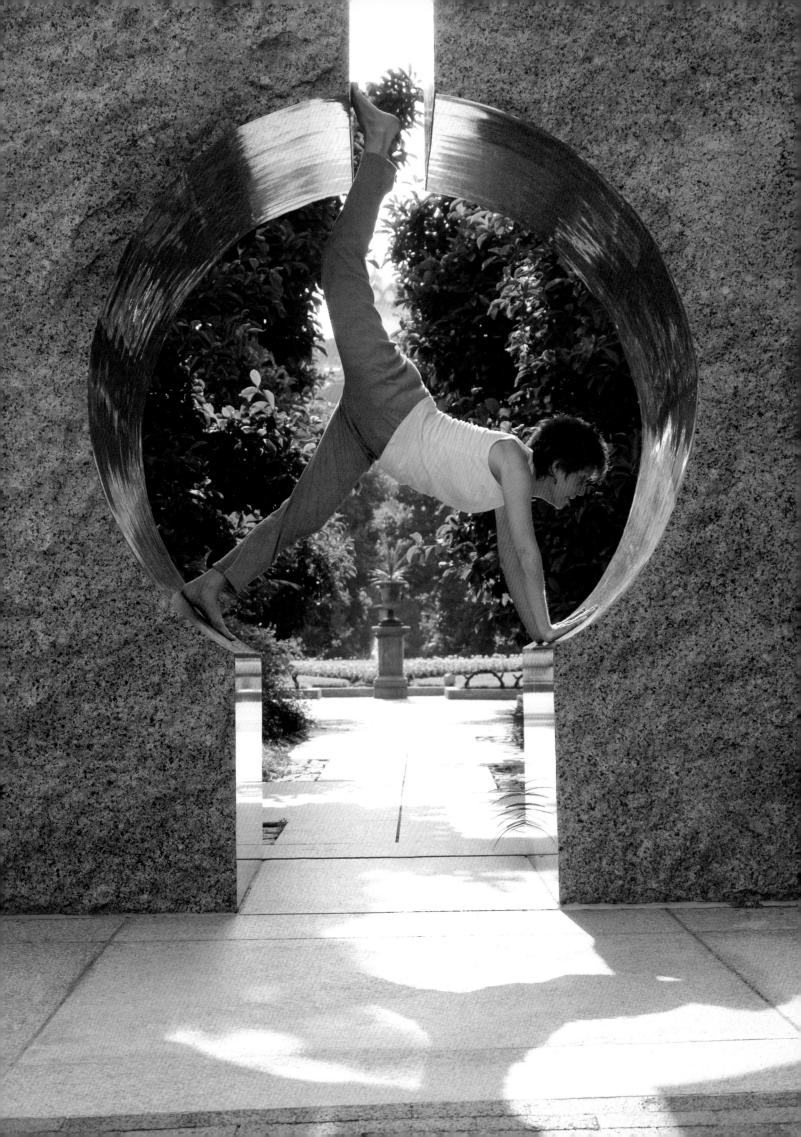

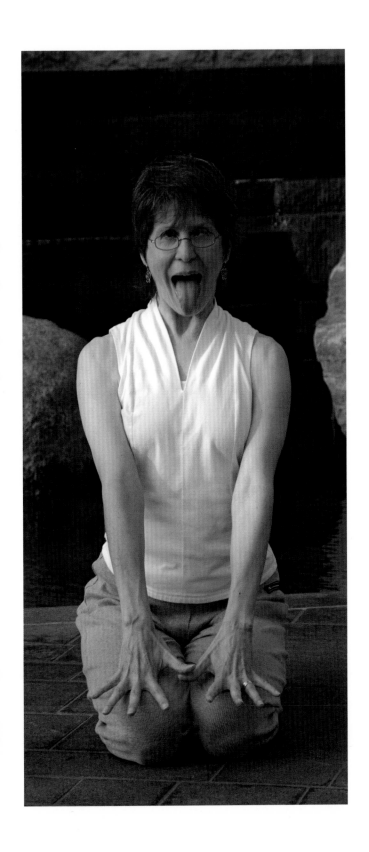

The freedom Karen found in stillness sustained her emotionally and spiritually through the treatment of her ovarian cancer. The shock of the diagnosis "heightened my awareness of the importance of breath as the foundation of life and a fundamental component of yoga," she says. Her chemotherapy and ultimate hysterectomy "could not have gone more smoothly. The yoga prepared me mentally and physically and I received so much support from my yoga friends that I recovered quickly from the surgery."

Cancer taught Karen that complete control over one's life is an illusion. Yoga taught her how to cope with that startling reality. "Thanks to yoga I'm calmer and much more open," says Karen, "and at 53, I'm finally accessing my own power which means, paradoxically, unclenching my grip." She says yoga enables her to express herself honestly because "it helps me tame my controlling ego." Karen has come to realize that "the ability to make appropriate choices comes from being fully present, open to creative inspiration and free to flow with changing circumstances."

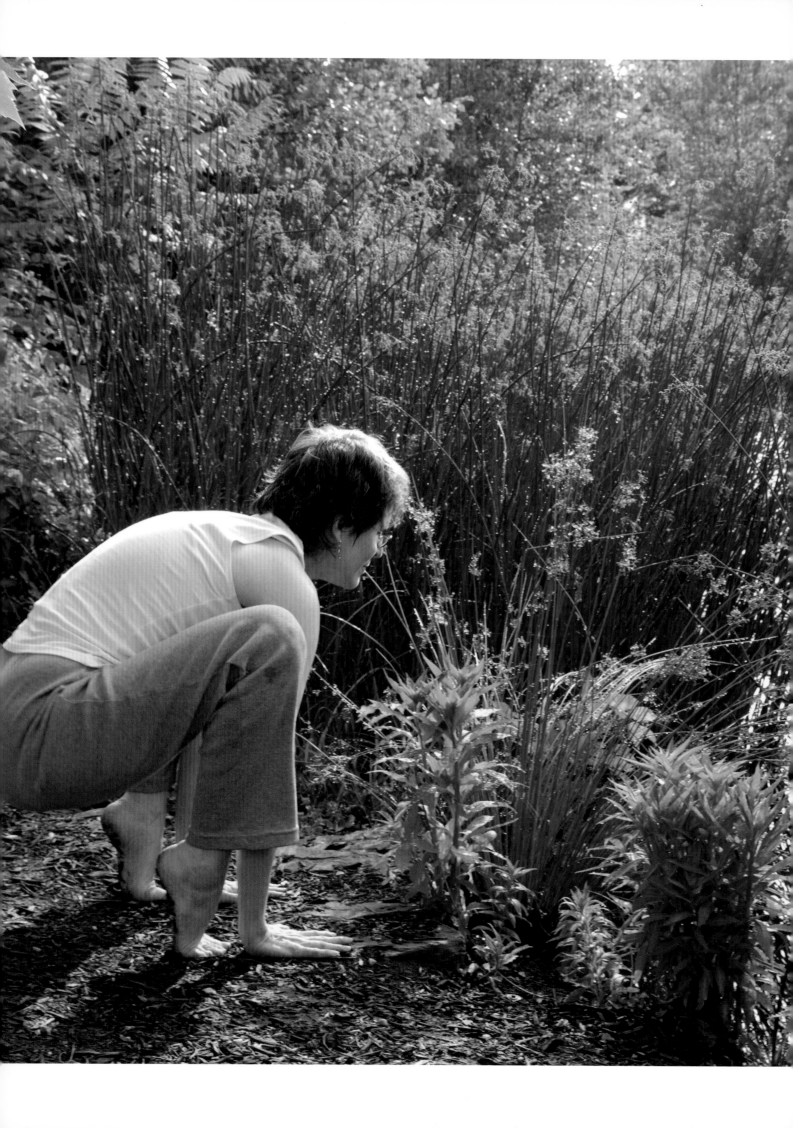

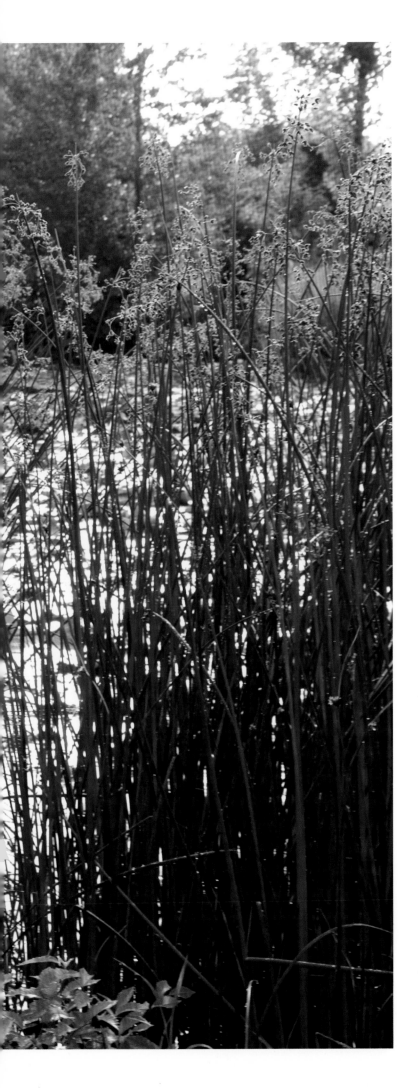

ABOUT KAREN

AGE	*53*
PROFESSION	*Executive coach*
TYPE OF PRACTICE	*Hatha yoga*
LEVEL OF EXPERIENCE	*8 years*
GREATEST BENEFIT OF THE PRACTICE TO KAREN	*Physical well-being & flexibility*
KAREN'S ADVICE TO OTHERS	*Don't get involved in what you think yoga should be. Just show up and relax into it and you'll enjoy some surprises.*

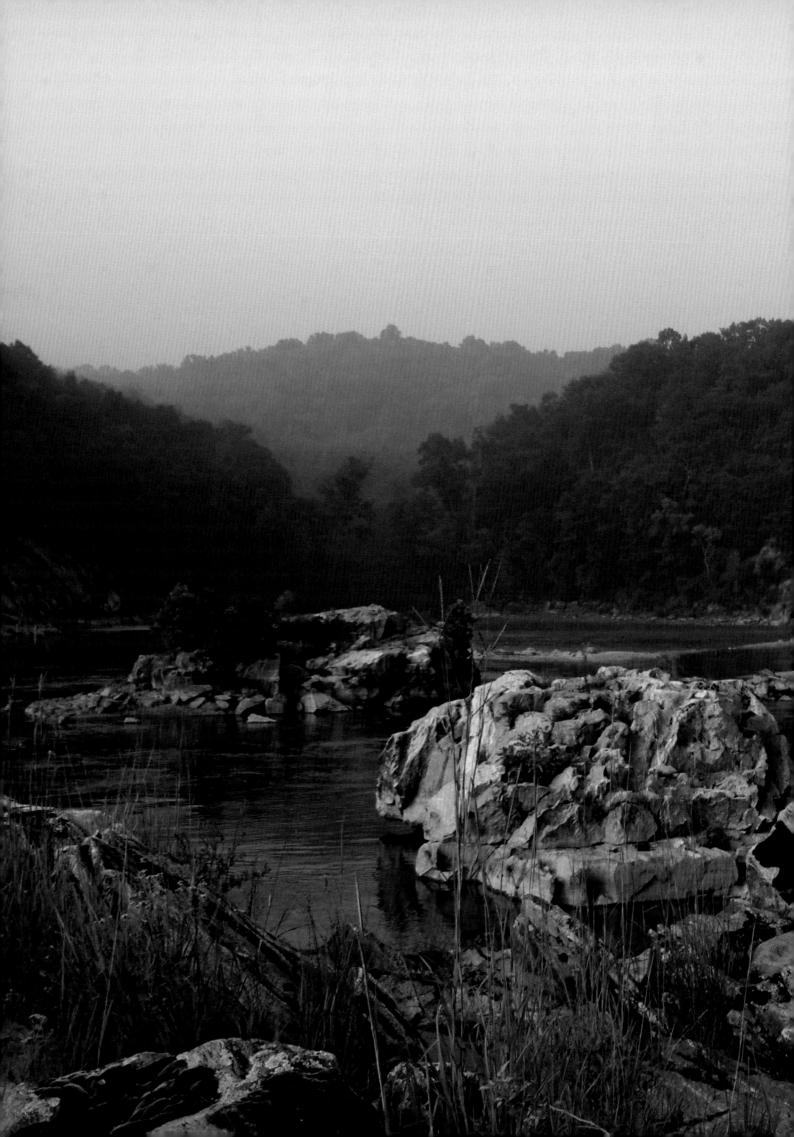

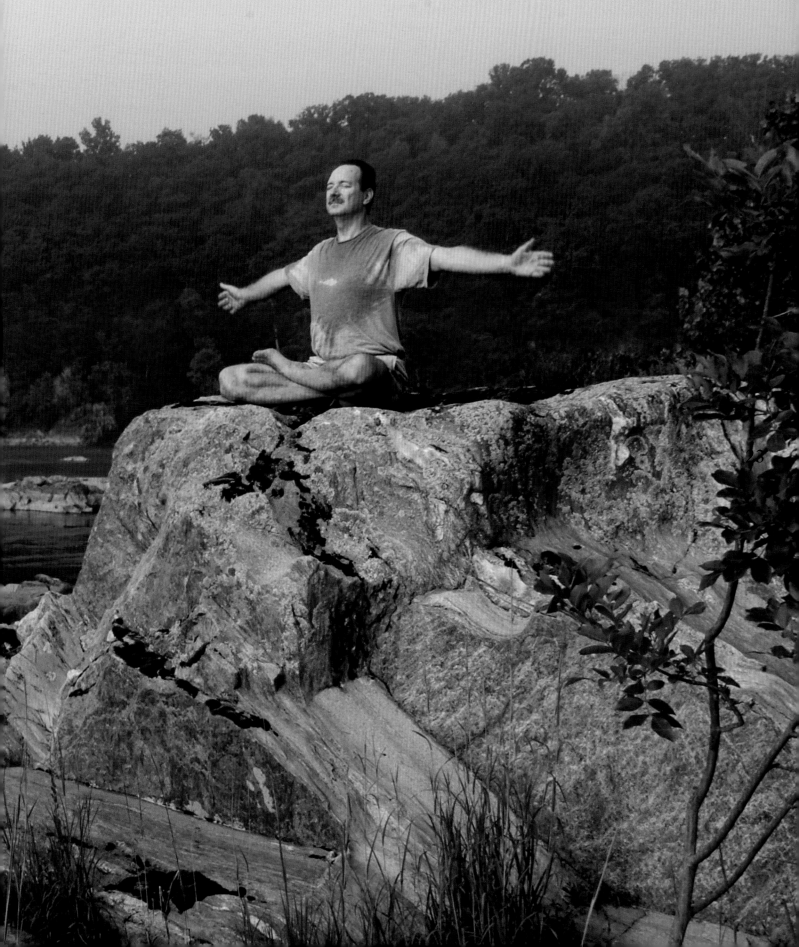

WILL

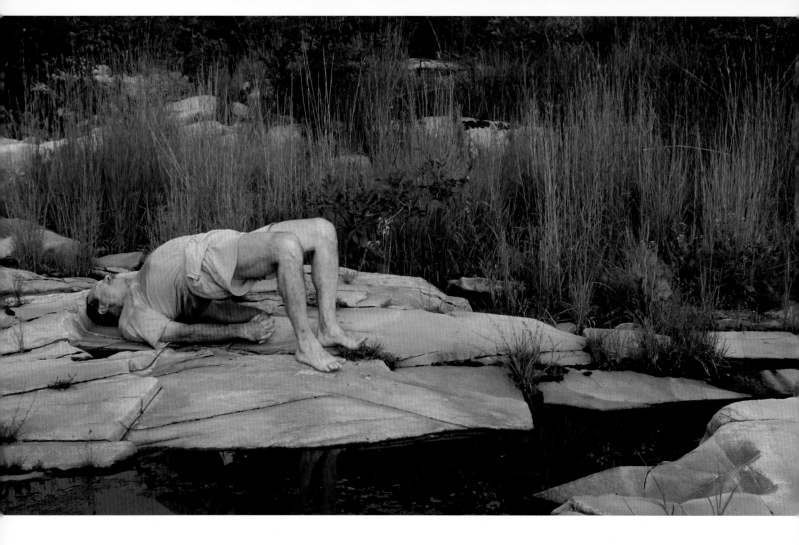

WILL CAME TO YOGA AT THE AGE OF 60,

an engineer and former competitive athlete, seeking balance in his life. Early retirement after 35 years of environmental engineering and policy management and the onset of a new career dovetailed with the loss of both of his parents and the launching of his two children into careers of their own. Many of the familiar pillars of his life were crumbling.

Adding to Will's apprehension, "The world was becoming less secure," with increasing political tensions at home and around the globe and with accelerating environmental change. He felt the need to do something but found he was caught in a pattern of "alternating between anxiety and numbness." He can't say for certain why he turned to yoga just that it felt like a "gravitational pull" toward the promise of "balance and centering of mind, body and spirit ... whatever that meant."

Little did Will know that yoga would provide him with a balanced life by throwing him off center. After years of competitive basketball and the competitive work environment, Will found it difficult to turn his focus inward where he would inevitably encounter the multiple voices of his internal dialogue, at times prideful, judging, berating, even boastful but never silent. He learned that his incessant inner chatter robbed him of a full and rich appreciation of life's precious moments. "I admit to being a reforming sufferer of awareness deficit disorder," he says in wry recognition.

Will quickly came to appreciate the concept of "the edge" in his yoga practice. In yoga, an edge is both a place of discomfort and the body's way of communicating the need for caution. "Working to improve balance at all levels required the counterintuitive approach

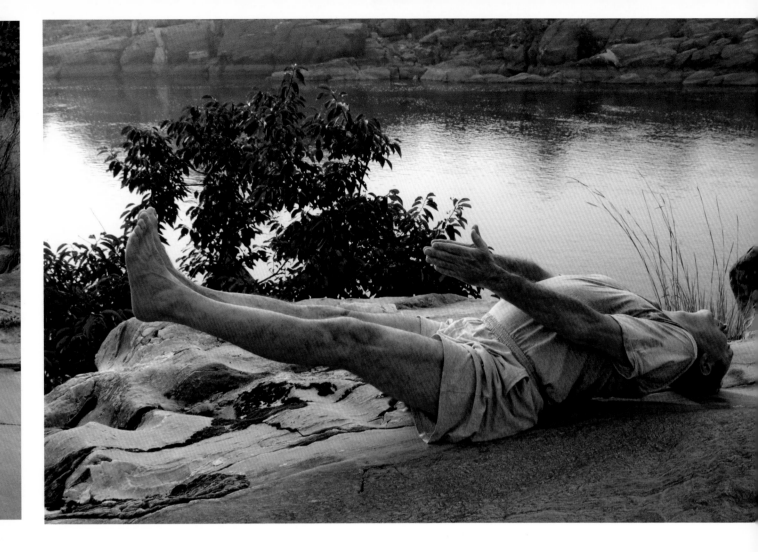

of constantly finding edges and working within them, not pushing through them," Will explains. "Learning to put aside a competitive approach allowed me to listen to my body respectfully but it also presented emotional and spiritual edges that were entirely new to me. I came to acknowledge the natural feelings of insecurity of being a beginner. I learned to chuckle at my ego when I was the only male in class and all the women were advancing faster than me. Most importantly, I realized that I could practice awareness of my edges outside of the studio with an attitude of acceptance and compassion."

The introduction of a new and unexpected edge came for Will when he accepted the invitation to step outside the disciplined environment of the yoga studio to experiment with a spontaneous, playful, creative practice outdoors. The idea appealed to him and he felt extremely comfortable in the rocky, riverside environment he had chosen.

His yoga practice "off the mat" went smoothly as long as he stayed within the bounds of traditional poses. When prompted to improvise, Will froze. He wondered, "How could I spontaneously depart from millennia-old guidance?" His inner dialogue pumped up the volume, "I'm not creative. I'll look like a fugitive from an exercise class in Sun City!" And then it happened. Awareness. Hearing his internal chatter, feeling his discomfort, Will recognized that he was experiencing an edge. He breathed. He chuckled. He relaxed ... and suddenly, "I was gone," he says. "There was nothing but the moment. I was in balance on an edge with no dimensions."

Will is no longer caught in the inertia of his anxiety. His energy refueled, he is able to focus clearly on his new professional mission to design and build ecologically based water filtration and delivery systems. He embraces the many complex challenges of his life by applying the principles of yoga.

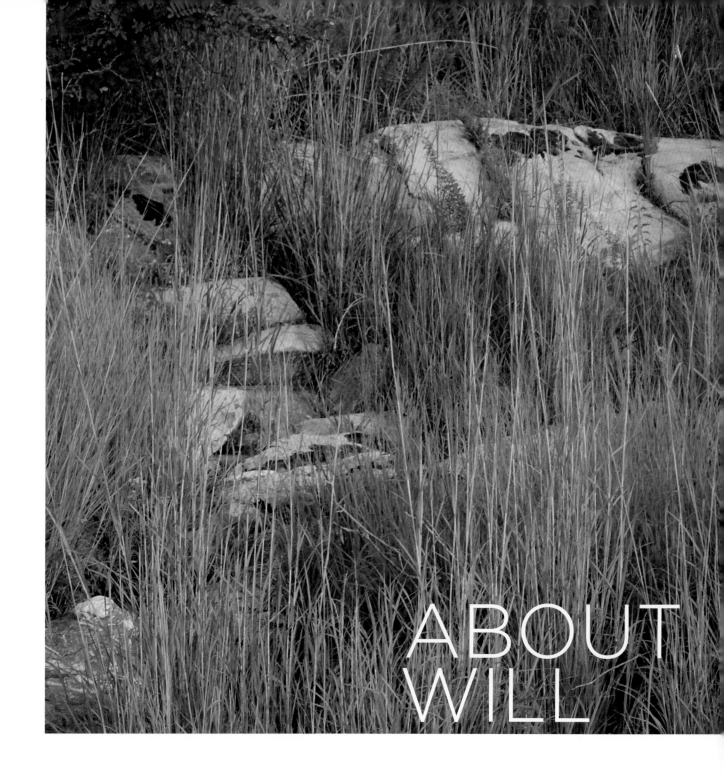

ABOUT WILL

AGE	*60*
PROFESSION	*Executive V.P. and Sustainable Water Filtration Engineer*
TYPE OF PRACTICE	*Hatha, Ashtanga (Power Yoga)*
LEVEL OF EXPERIENCE	*Beginner*
GREATEST BENEFIT OF THE PRACTICE TO WILL	*Learning about physical, emotional and spiritual edges. Yoga teaches that balance is achieved neither in retreating from nor pushing through edges. It comes from finding ways to soften into them thereby expanding one's sphere of comfort.*

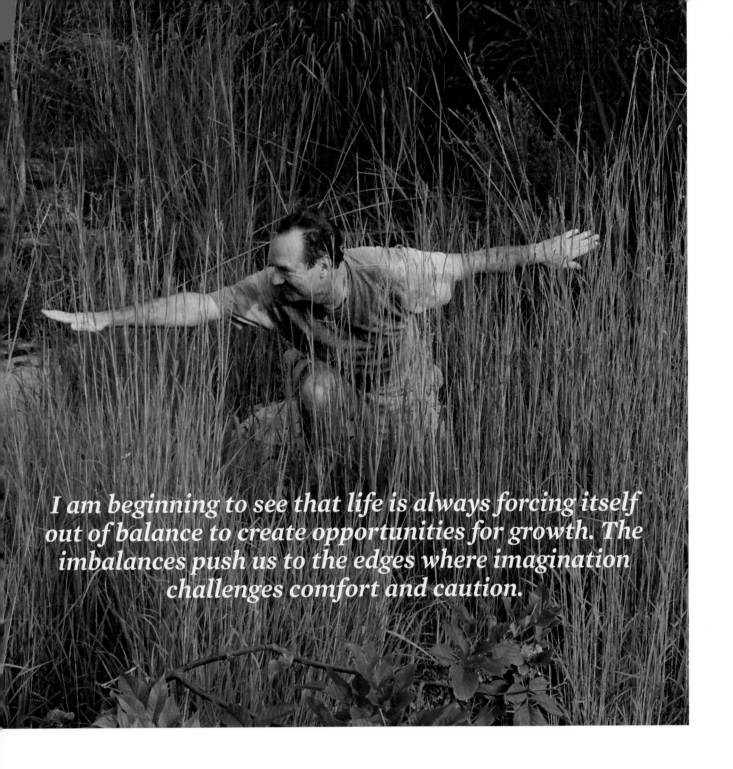

I am beginning to see that life is always forcing itself out of balance to create opportunities for growth. The imbalances push us to the edges where imagination challenges comfort and caution.

WILL'S ADVICE
TO OTHERS

Embrace your edges! Not respecting edges leads to injury, retreating from them brings stagnation. Explore the edge of taking your yoga off your mat and take what you learn creatively into the world.

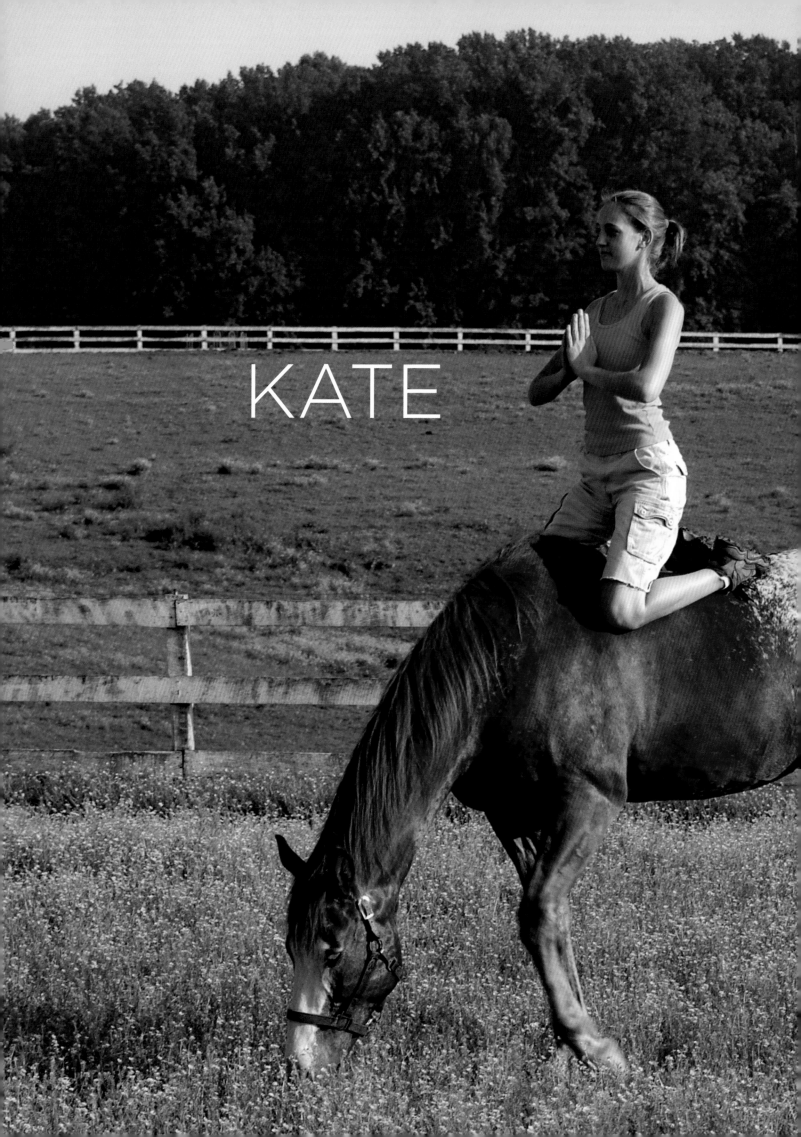

KATE

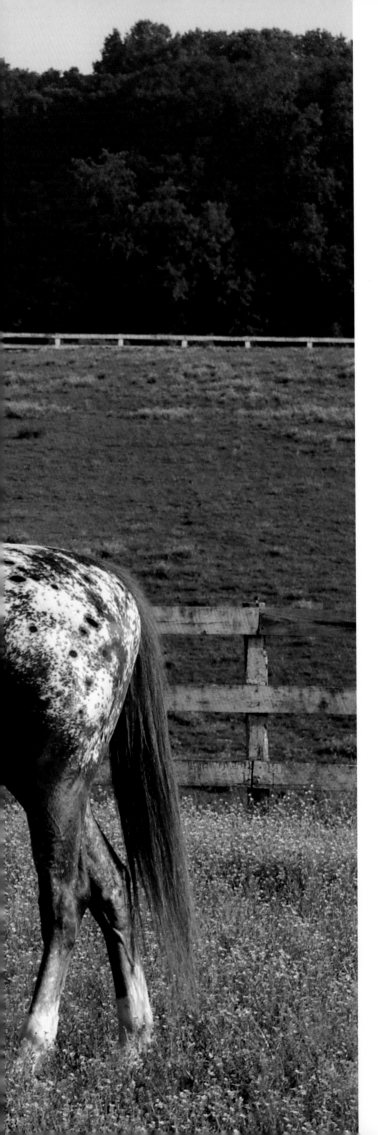

KATE, AT 17, HAS BEEN DOING YOGA FOR, WELL, 17 YEARS.

"Since yoga, to me, is wholly integrated into life and my mom practiced yoga when she was pregnant with me, I can truthfully say that I don't know life without yoga."

Kate describes her yoga as "environment inspired" as she incorporates it into her daily activities, seamlessly blending chores, studies, sports and creative play with the basics of the practice ... breath, focus and flow. "Yoga, on the mat, is something I come back to now and then to remind me about proper alignment in classic poses and to help me manage my scoliosis. But for me, yoga is about how I interact with the world."

A favorite part of Kate's world is a field laden in spring with buttercups where her horse, John, loves to luxuriate. Kate says that her lifelong experience with yoga helps her to feel trusting and playful on horseback. She loves the freedom, for herself and for John, of riding bareback. And the rolling green hills beside his stable evoke an ancient, mystical setting in which her imagination soars. She and John are best friends and heroic adventurers. After a long afternoon of saving lives and ensuring justice, they return to their lovely field of buttercups to bask in the sun.

While it's challenging for Kate to come to her mat for a traditional, disciplined yoga routine, she realizes that symptoms of her scoliosis "drastically reduce when I consistently practice." And, she says, "no matter how bogged down I get in my mind or body, a good yoga-ing makes me feel right as rain."

29

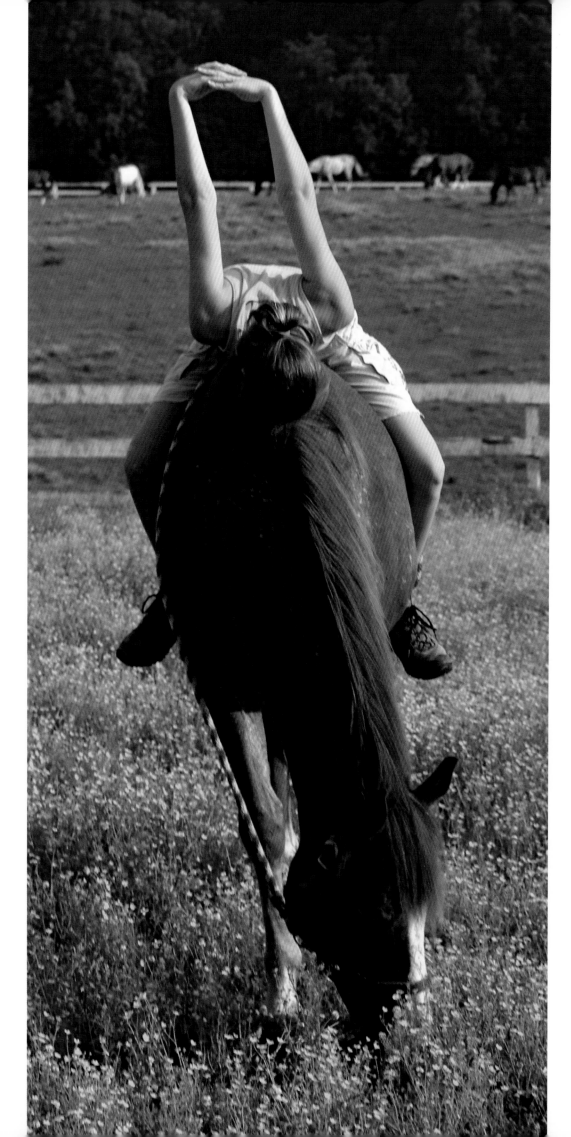

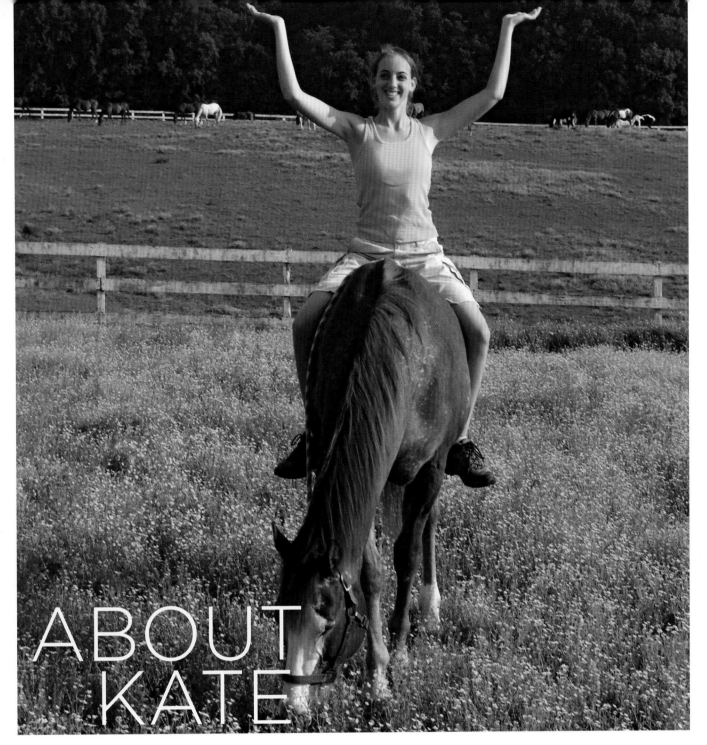

ABOUT KATE

AGE	*17*
PROFESSION	*High school student*
TYPE OF PRACTICE	*Environment-inspired creative yoga*
LEVEL OF EXPERIENCE	*A lifer*
GREATEST BENEFIT OF THE PRACTICE TO KATE	*It helps reduce the effects of my scoliosis and relaxes my mind and body when I'm feeling stressed.*
KATE'S ADVICE TO OTHERS	*Go out and play. When you take the risk to get off your mat your mind and body will open to surprising benefits. If you're self-conscious, grab a friend and a camera and go to your favorite place where no one else is, and then just play. Challenge each other to be the best embodiment of a tree, a gazelle, a puddle of goo ... anything and everything you can think of. You'll have a lot of fun and be better friends for it. Anyone who happens by will probably be inspired.*

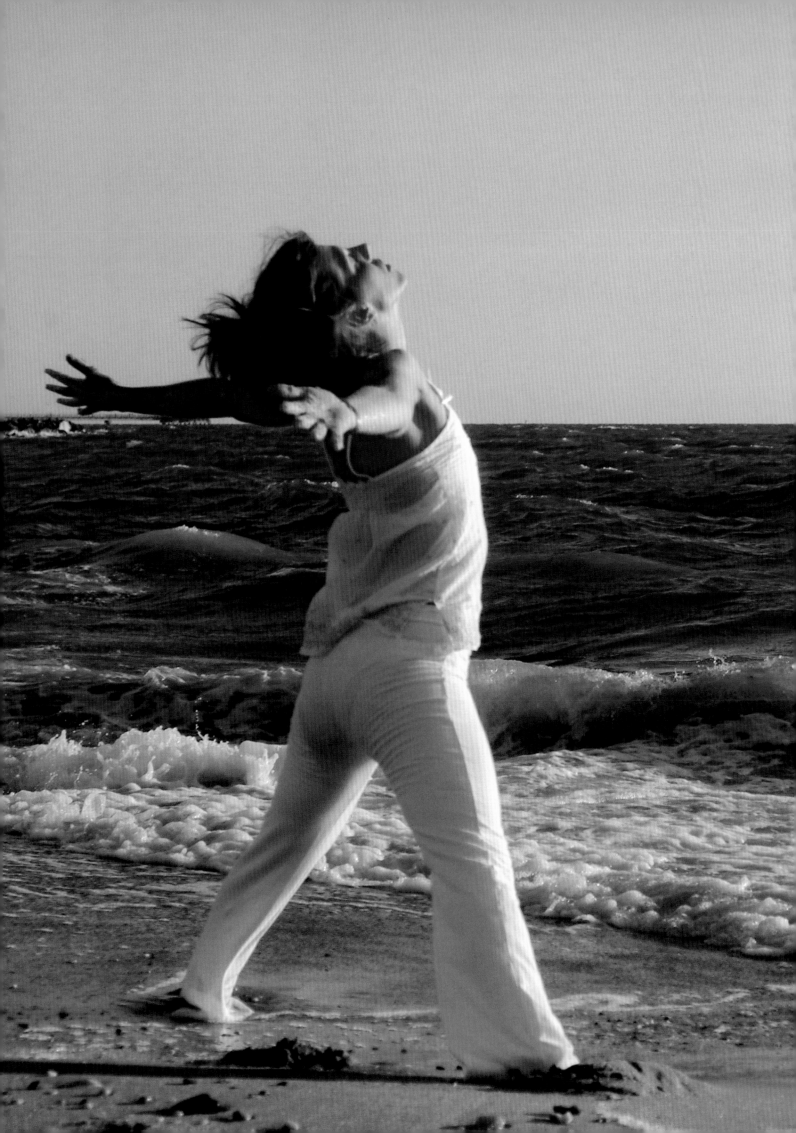

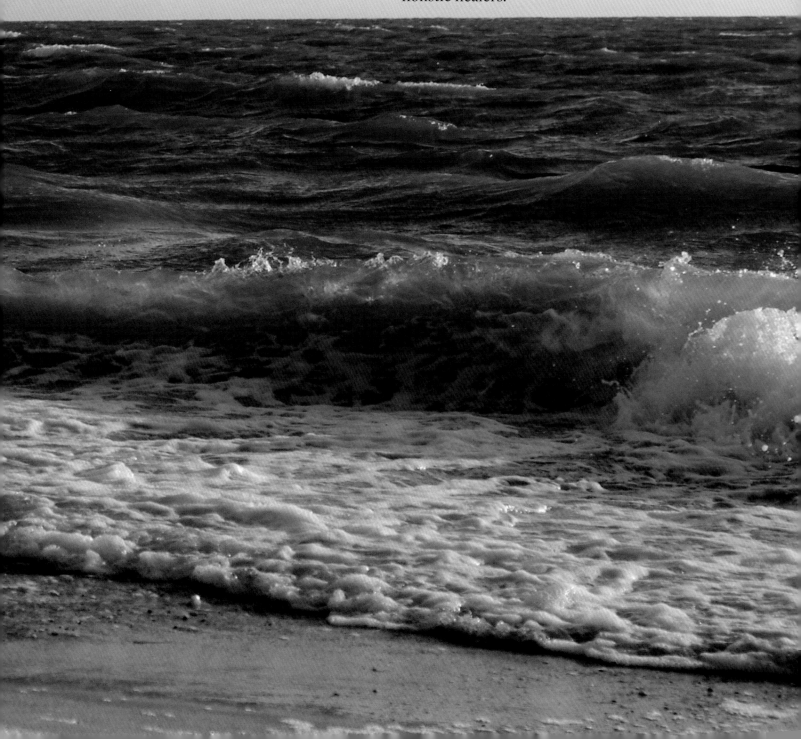

COURTNEY

COURTNEY, AT AGE 26, THREE MONTHS AFTER THE BIRTH OF HER DAUGHTER, was diagnosed with Hodgkin's Disease. Her life became a frantic search for treatments that might save her life and allow her to mother the child she'd just brought into the world. She tried mainstream medical procedures, changes in diet and the help of holistic healers.

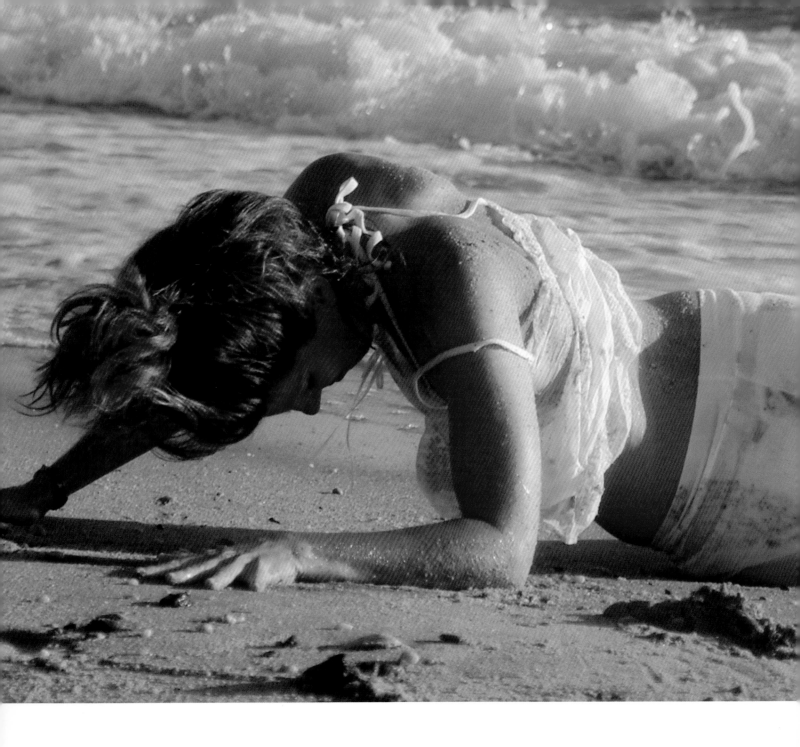

"My life was a wreck," she says. "I was living in terror and confusion." But she survived, and her daughter thrived—although not her marriage—and she began another search ... for peace and stability for them both. While the spectre of Hodgkin's disease may cast a faint shadow in Courtney's life, she's currently healthy and after 12 years of annual testing she is now considered cured. It was the upheaval of the dissolution of her marriage that left a more permanent mark.

A private yoga session and the classes that followed helped her find "a calm place inside myself" where, she says, she discovered "I am not my pain, or my fear. I am alive and well and it's alright."

"Yoga is like the ocean. When you're floating on the surface you can hear all the sounds of the beach. Kids squealing. Waves crashing. Birds squawking," says Courtney, now age 38. "But if you drop beneath the surface, it all quiets down. The deeper you go the more stillness

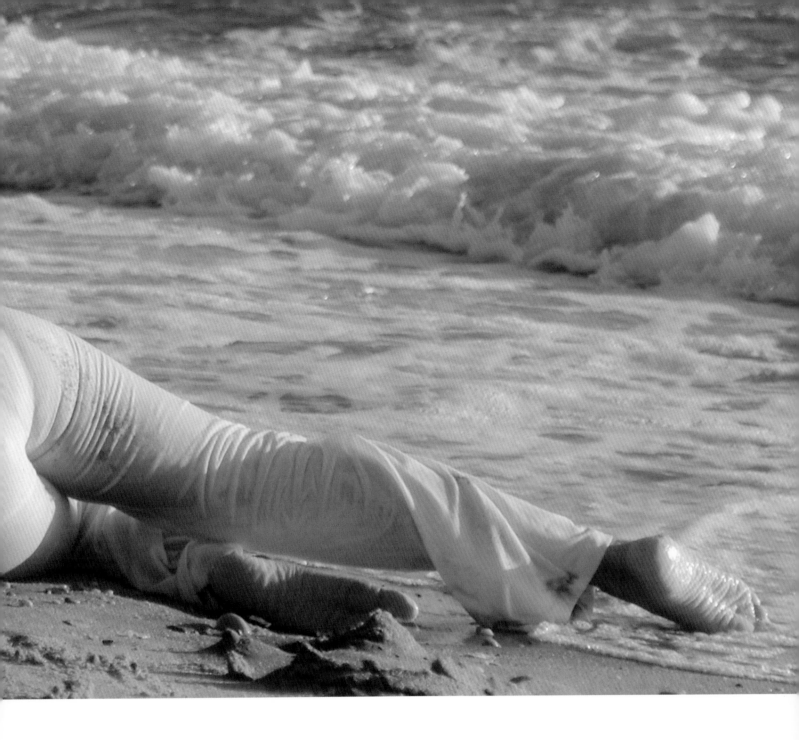

there is. Beneath all the noise and chaos you find total bliss." Courtney says her practice of yoga strengthened her mind, body and spirit. Her chronic confusion yielded to a newly found confidence that made such a difference in her life that she became a yoga teacher.

"I'm devoted to bringing yoga's benefits to others who need it," she says. "I especially like teaching teenagers because I can relate to their vulnerability and uncertainty."

While she believes in establishing a disciplined practice of yoga, grounded in proper alignment, inner awareness, good breathing techniques and the knowledge of classic poses, she says "the real magic happens when you free yourself of all the 'shoulds' and trust what your body knows."

Courtney joyfully creates her own yoga by uniting with her environment. "When I release myself to the moment and feel I am the ocean, the wind, the sand, and sky," she says, "I'm blissful and free—yes, that's the word ... free."

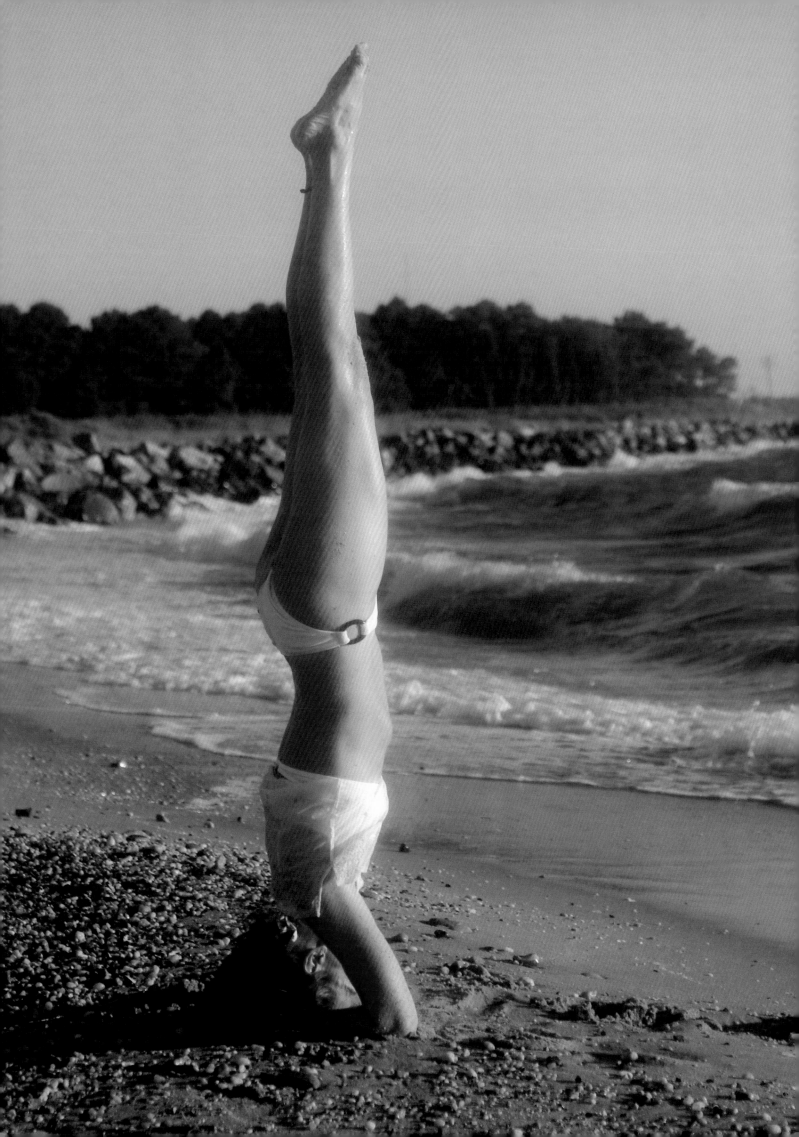

ABOUT COURTNEY

AGE	*38*
PROFESSION	*Full-time mom & part-time yoga instructor*
TYPE OF PRACTICE	*Hatha & Kundalini Yoga*
LEVEL OF EXPERIENCE	*Certified Hatha and Kundalini Yoga teacher*
GREATEST BENEFIT OF THE PRACTICE TO COURTNEY	*Feeling centered and calm regardless of what's going on around me; excellent health, improved strength, flexibility and self-assurance.*
COURTNEY'S ADVICE TO OTHERS	*Find a great teacher and learn the basics. Once you've mastered the fundamentals, free yourself of the rules and discover the bliss of uniting with your surroundings.*

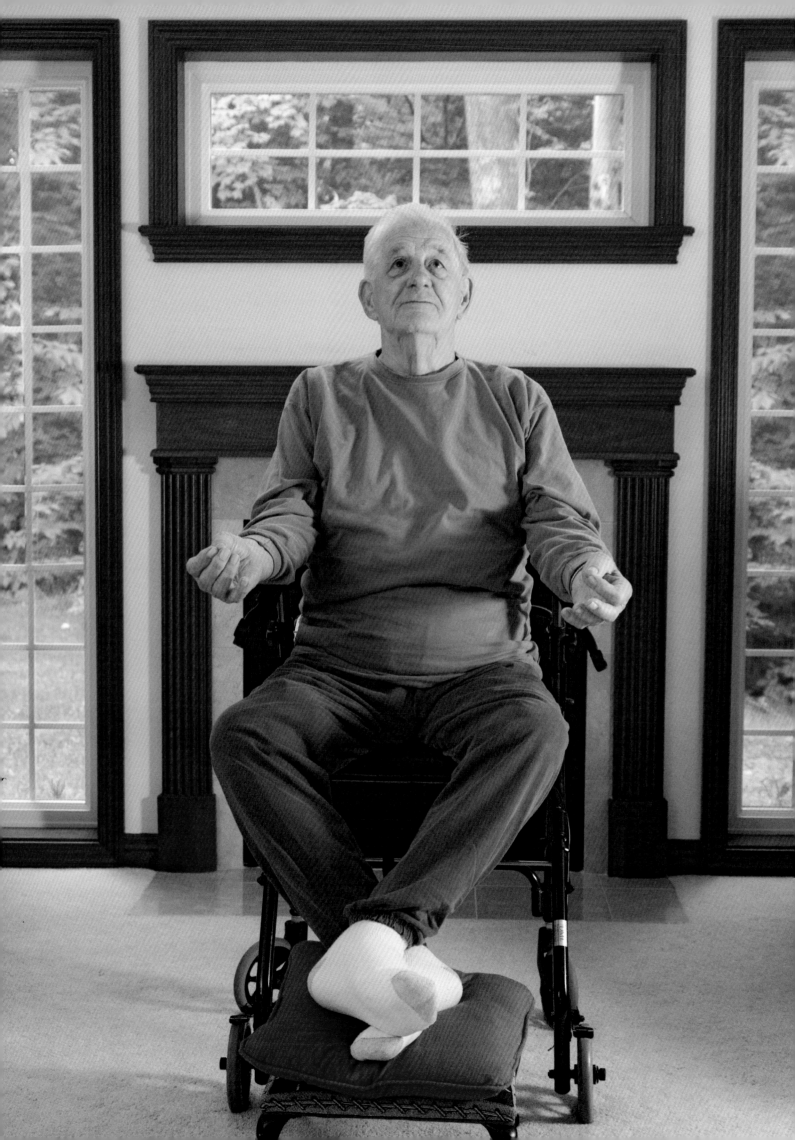

JOHN, AN 82-YEAR-OLD RETIRED GRAPHIC ARTIST and painter, had emergency open-heart surgery. Five weeks later he was practicing yoga for the first time in his life as part of his physical therapy regimen.

"After the surgery I would tire easily" and just walking made him feel light-headed and wobbly, says John. Yoga helped him regain his balance and stamina. It also helped him fend off post-surgical depression. Using a walker made him feel "my days were numbered and I was haunted by age-old regrets," he says. Yoga provided a way for the newly vulnerable John to manage his emotions and gave him a sense of "being in control of my own fate, if only for brief moments at a time."

"I could feel myself getting physically and emotionally stronger," he says. "I came to accept and even feel grateful for my wheels. With the yoga, I was able to see the walker as a tool for rehabilitation. I could even get creative with it so it brought some fun to the physical therapy."

Yoga also helped heal his relationship with his daughter, a yoga teacher from whom he'd been estranged since her adolescence. She visited him for the first time in more than a decade after his surgery and John smiles as he says, "I wouldn't have done any of this without her. She says her yoga helped her to let go of old resentments and put our past struggles behind her and it was her idea for me to try it." John says, "I will always be grateful that yoga brought us back together and helped me to open my heart to her." His smile returns, "Now that's an open-heart procedure you can't get from a surgeon."

JOHN

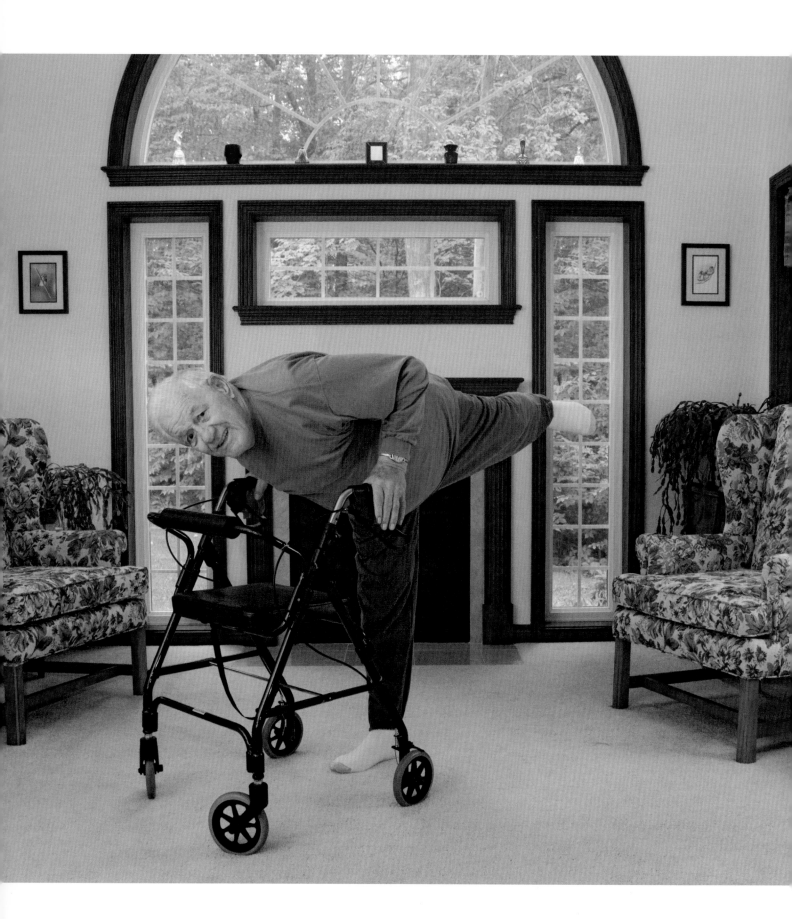

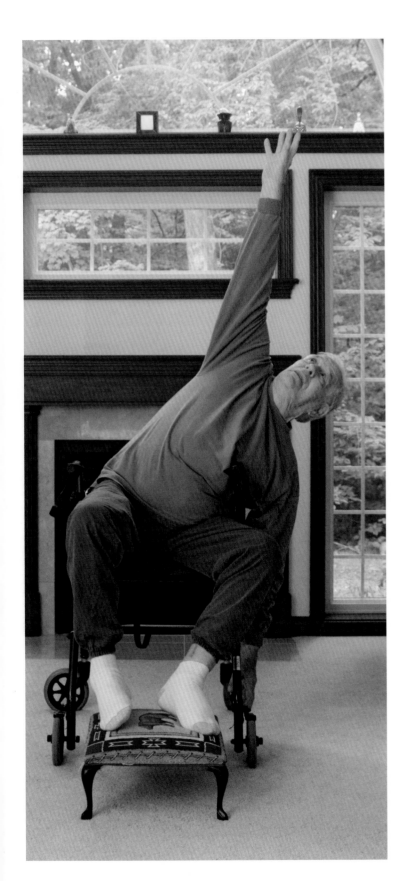

ABOUT JOHN

AGE	*82*
PROFESSION	*Retired graphic artist and painter*
TYPE OF PRACTICE	*Therapeutic yoga*
LEVEL OF EXPERIENCE	*Complete beginner*
GREATEST BENEFIT OF THE PRACTICE TO JOHN	*Stamina, balance, loving connection*
JOHN'S ADVICE TO OTHERS	*Do yoga, no matter what shape you're in. Find a good teacher and learn the right way to do it. Then let yourself have fun with it.*

41

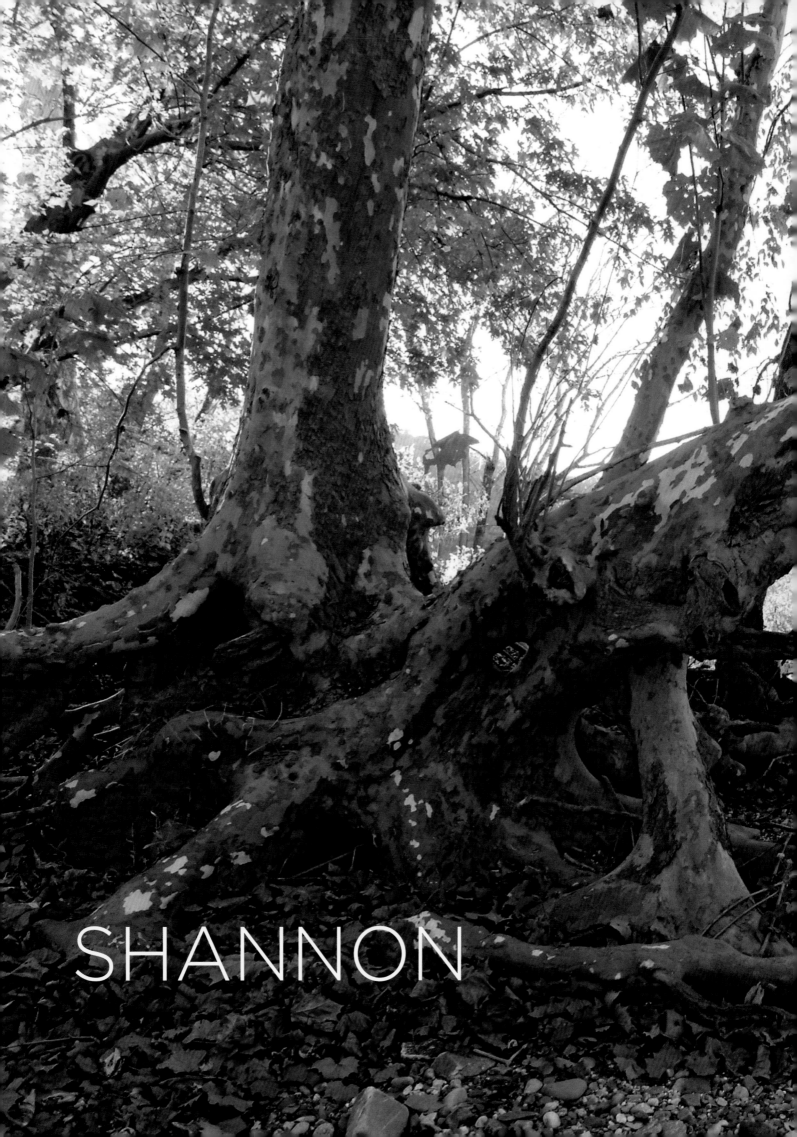

SHANNON

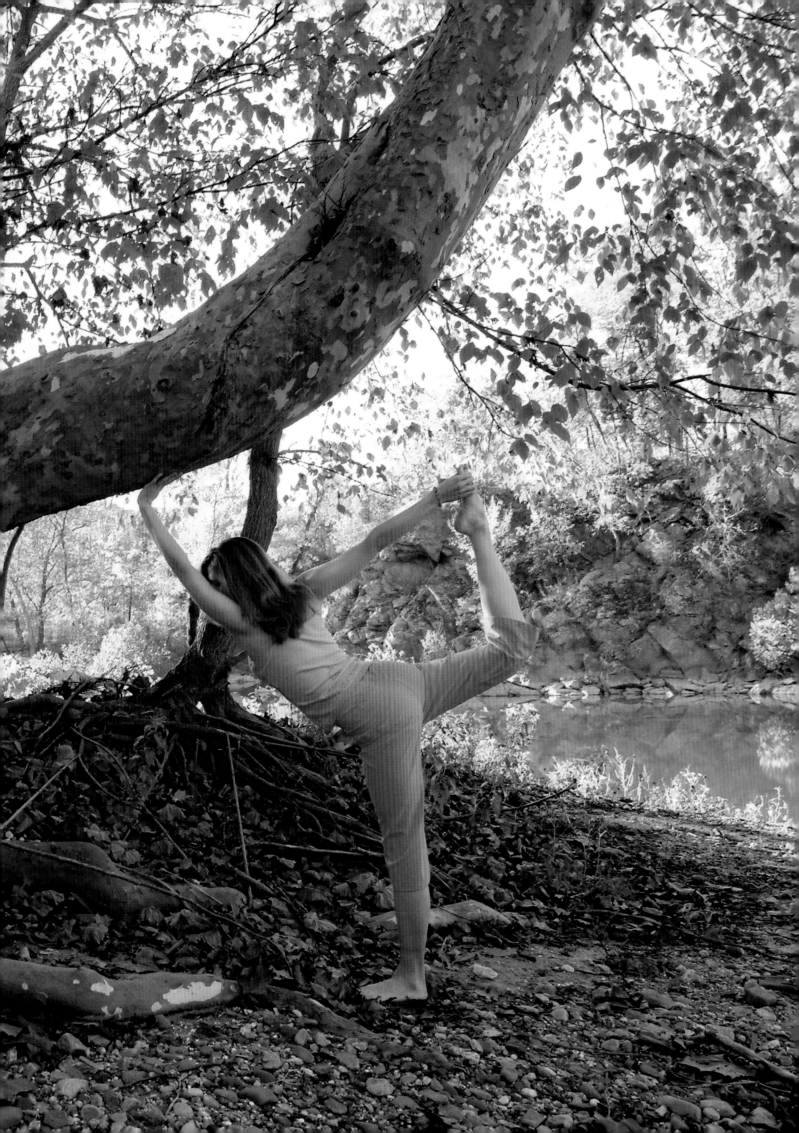

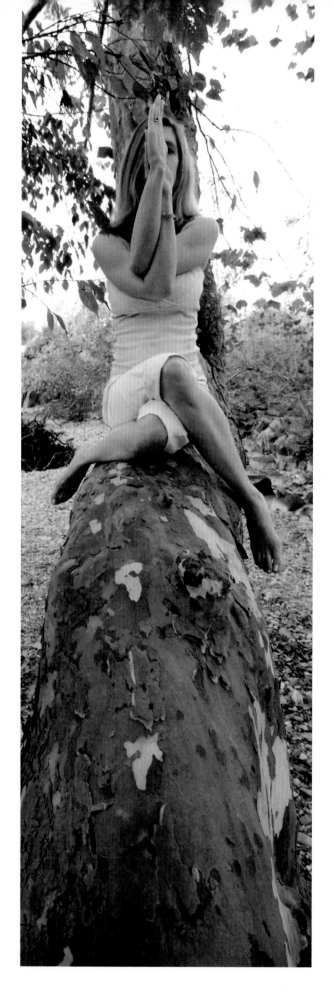

SOME OF SHANNON'S EARLIEST AND HAPPIEST MEMORIES INVOLVE THE PLAYFUL practice of yoga. Her mother practiced on the living room floor and would invite her "to stretch my body like a snake or strike the pose of a roaring lion." So, at 35, Shannon, an education research and development professional, was delighted to rekindle the magic of those childhood days by literally going out on a limb. She chose to create her yoga around a huge sycamore tree where she became a tree goddess and found her roots at a river's edge.

There was a time when Shannon had lost her sense of play. She was living in New York City, cramming into the subway each day, eating on the fly and feeling overwhelmed. She began suffering severe abdominal pains that eluded medical diagnosis. Shannon realized that she had to find a way to reduce her stress. She consulted with a nutritionist and joined a yoga class. The first time she entered the studio she "felt a sense of peace that put me on the path of self-healing." She learned that through yoga she could quiet her mind enough to "relax the smooth muscles of my gut, ending the cycle of pain" that had dominated her life for more than a year.

Shannon continued practicing and found that she was able to manage the stress of changing jobs, relocating, marrying and giving birth to a daughter, all while improving her strength, balance and flexibility. She says, "Yoga led me to positive lifestyle changes as I learned what it meant to be physically, emotionally and spiritually healthy."

Shannon's desire to share these benefits with others led her to enroll in yoga teacher training. She has come full circle, teaching parents to practice yoga with their babies and toddlers. "New parents can feel crushed under unexpected pressures and uncertainty," Shannon says. "If I can help them feel centered and calm and teach them to practice yoga playfully with their little ones, I feel as though I'm honoring the excellent mothering that I enjoyed."

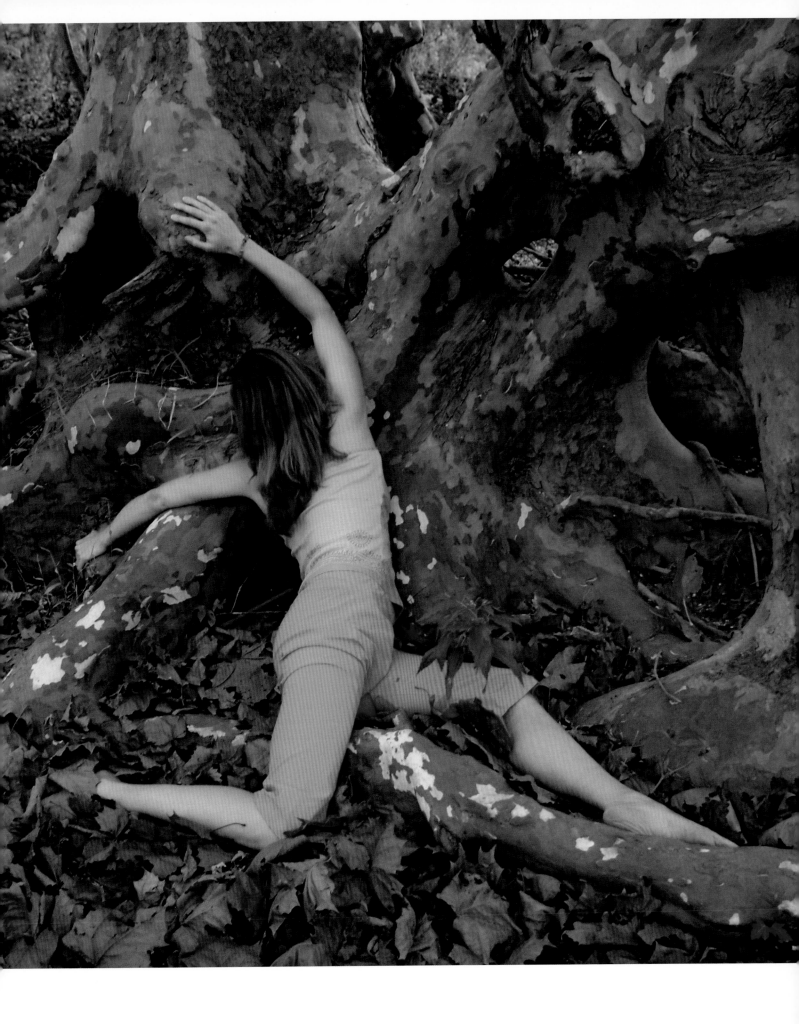

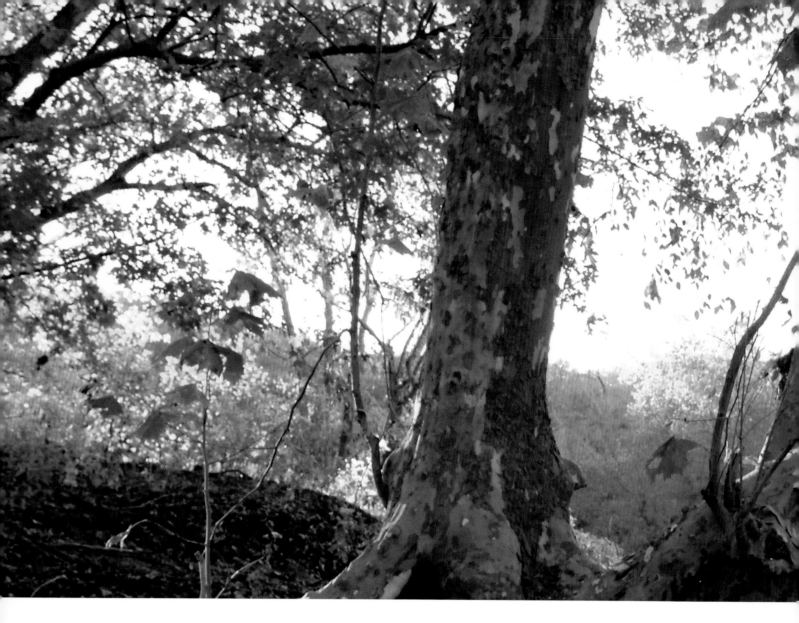

ABOUT SHANNON

AGE	*35*
PROFESSION	*Education Research & Development; Part-time Yoga Teacher*
TYPE OF PRACTICE	*Hatha*
LEVEL OF EXPERIENCE	*8 years*
GREATEST BENEFIT OF THE PRACTICE TO SHANNON	*Physical strengthening and improved balance and flexibility, along with stress reduction and the ability to activate self-healing.*
SHANNON'S ADVICE TO OTHERS	*Have patience with yourself and your practice. Many of the benefits of yoga are realized gradually. Flexibility, for example, can sneak up on you. It may be that you need props at first, to sit in certain positions or to accomplish a particular pose. Then, one day, you may be surprised to find that you don't need the props at all.*

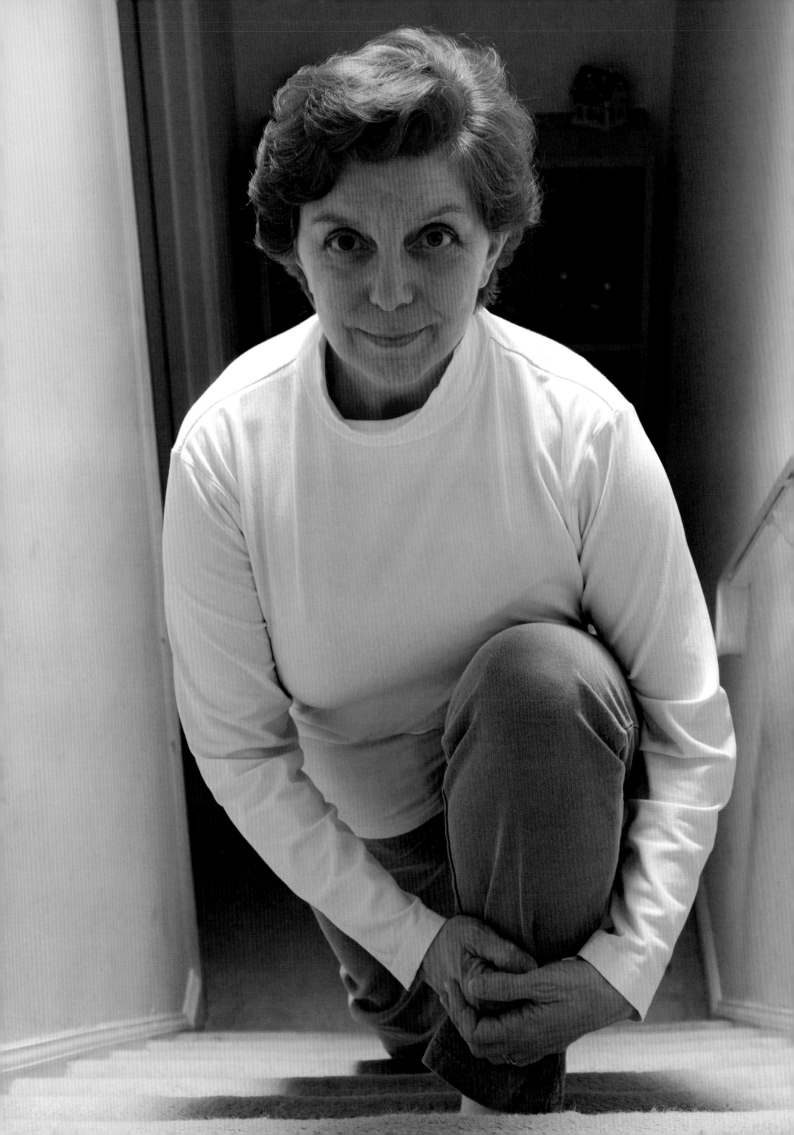

BEBA HAS HER HANDS FULL. The 55-year-old scientist, seamstress, stained-glass artist, wife and mother spends several hours a day running upstairs and down. A devoted and meticulous homemaker, Beba insists on doing all of the household chores even while managing several creative projects, including a scholarly book on Antarctica. When friends ask her how she does it all, she perks up and answers, "Yoga!"

Beba discovered yoga eight years ago when her daughter's boyfriend encouraged her to attend a class taught by his mom. She began with a gentle hatha yoga class and became a devotee after only one session. "The attunement I felt with my body on that first day was so powerful that I knew I would never want to stop," she says. Her enthusiasm made it easy for her to establish a daily home practice.

"I do not think about how to practice at home," Beba says. She has become adept at integrating yoga into her daily activities. After hours of research at the computer, for example, "My body tells me when I need to stretch and breathe deeply," she says. Almost without thought, she finds herself "reaching up, readjusting my spine, making space in my ribcage so my breath flows easily. Then my mind and body relax together."

Sewing, one of Beba's favorite endeavors,

can be punishing to the spine. For Beba, though, "My body knows how to align itself so that I can get the job done and actually feel good, not sore or achy," and that goes for everything she does throughout her day "thanks to yoga." Beba's repeated trips up and down the stairs, once a burden, now offer an opportunity to engage in a playful, spontaneous practice. "On my way up my body is likely to go into a nice big lunge. Before I know it I've got one leg folded underneath me and the other stretched out behind. Because of my yoga practice, I know when the alignment is right. I don't have to analyze it. It's right when it feels perfect!"

Beba acknowledges that working at home all day can be emotionally draining but she has come to rely on her yoga practice to get her over the hump. "When I feel my energy dropping and my mood sliding," she says, "I know it's time to get up and move." A stretch might lead to a twist or a bend which "can put me in the mood for a more energetic release." It's then that Beba's traditional yoga poses transform into a more creative outlet. She plays some of her favorite Latin music and lets herself go. "I close my eyes and let my body stretch and sway." Yoga becomes a dance. "There is no mind, no body, nothing separate from anything else. It's all one," Beba says, "and that's my yoga!"

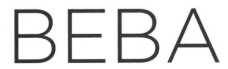

BEBA

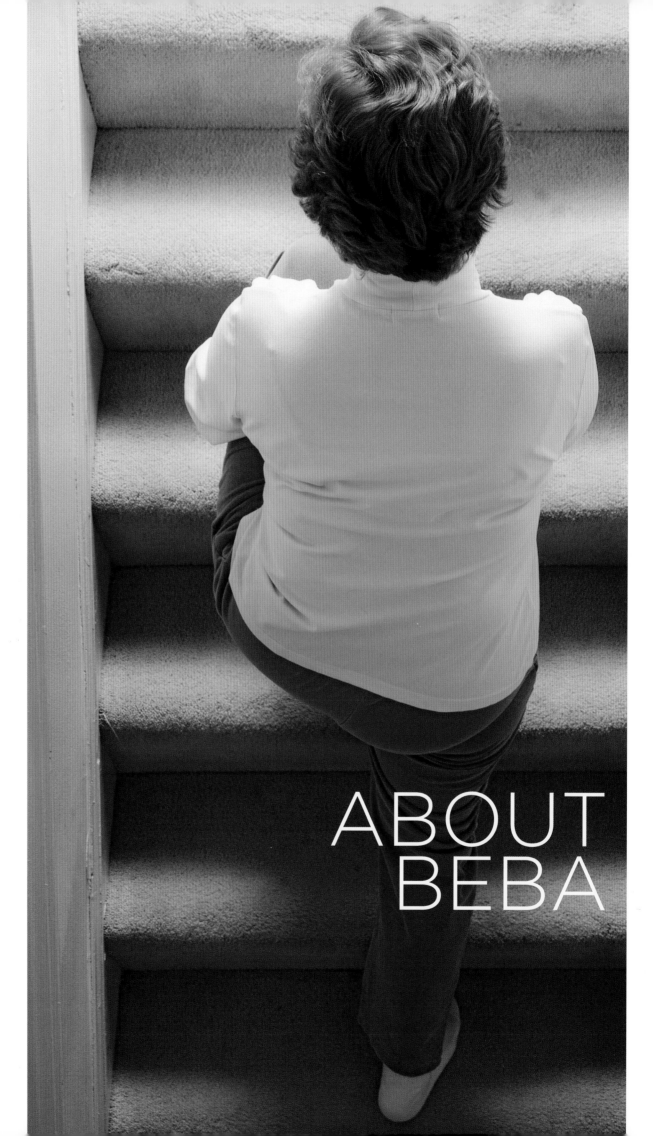

ABOUT
BEBA

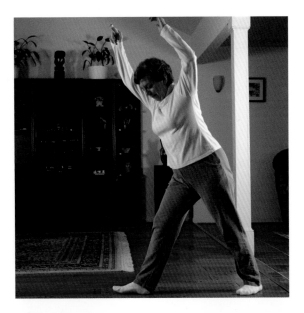
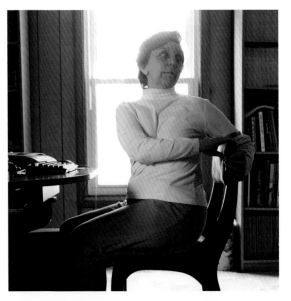
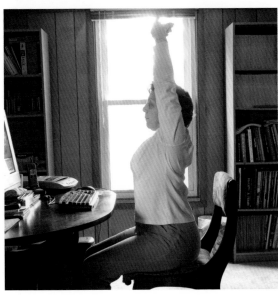
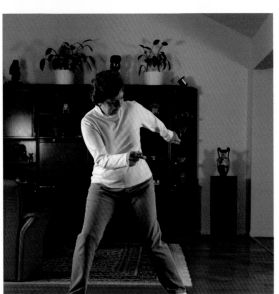

AGE *55*

PROFESSION *Homemaker, Scientist, Author*

TYPE OF PRACTICE *Fusion of yoga in daily activities, Hatha, Kundalini Yoga*

LEVEL OF EXPERIENCE *8 years*

GREATEST BENEFIT OF THE PRACTICE TO BEBA *It lifts my mood and keeps me strong and flexible. When I get tired, a yoga stretch or twist revives me and I can get things done.*

BEBA'S ADVICE TO OTHERS *Take a class to learn the right way to do the basic poses then bring your yoga into your daily life. Sneak it into the grocery store and to the post office. Practice breathing while you drive. Watch how yoga energizes your whole life!*

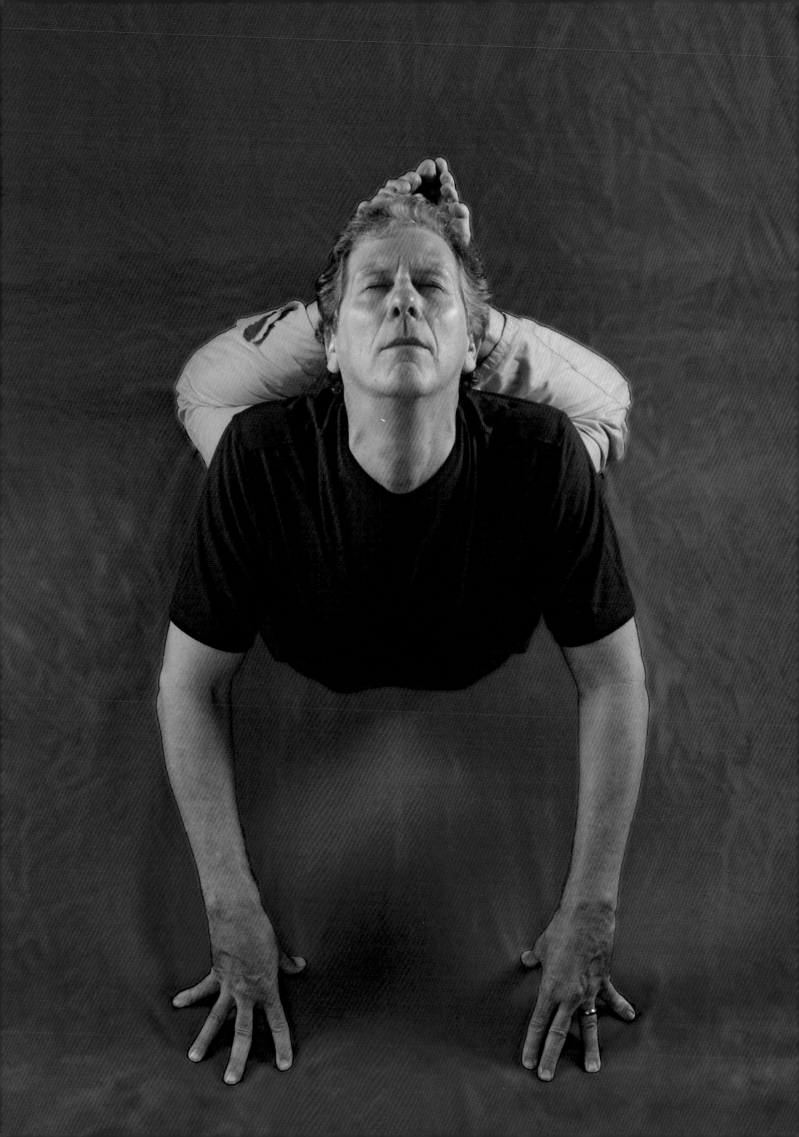

JUSTIN, AN INTROVERT, loves contra dancing, a pastime that looks like a hybrid of square dancing and the line dancing you might see in a country-western bar. It's vigorous and playful, the "perfect counterpoint" to the contemplative quality of his yoga practice. "Yoga is training for letting go," he says, "it keeps me from getting stuck in the ordinary stressors of everyday life and opens my heart to joyful interaction."

At 56, Justin, a security systems sales engineer, is an advanced yogi who has maintained a disciplined practice for more than 30 years. He began his study of yoga in the early 1970's when, like many of his contemporaries, he set out to explore altered states of consciousness. "It seemed to me that sensitizing the body was the place to start." Armed with Richard Hittleman's, "Introduction to Yoga" and Swami Vishnu-devananda's "The Complete Illustrated Book of Yoga," Justin embarked on what would become his life-long journey of self-discovery through yoga.

In the beginning, Justin practiced diligently for 60 to 90 minutes, four or five times a week. He followed the regimens recommended in the books and enrolled in a teacher-training course. Justin learned to follow his instincts regarding his practice and now devotes about 20 minutes each morning to pranayama (breathing techniques) and asana (postures.)

His morning practice allows him "to shake off who I think I am by dipping myself into the direct experience of life's flow ... enjoying the cascade of energy it produces. What is left behind is the stillness of simple witnessing, an allowing of experience to occur, unnamed."

That release led Justin to the dance floor. "Contra dancing, for me, is playful and powerful" in a way that is complemented by yoga. "Identity is lost within the act of dancing and the 'I' that remains is the ineffable vibrancy of pure existence." Justin reports that the boundaries between yoga, dancing, and life have happily blurred for him. "It's all one thing," he says, "who I am out of doing yoga is who I am on the dance floor and who I am in life."

JUSTIN

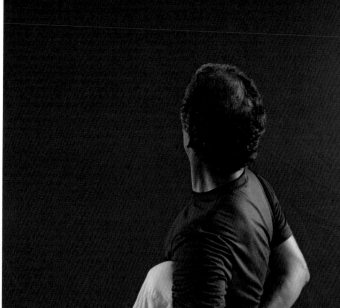

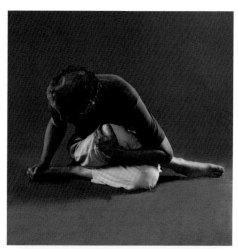

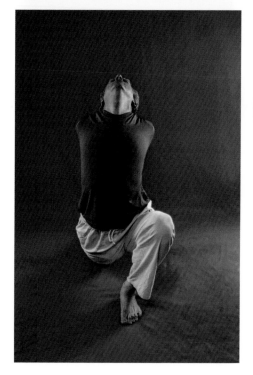

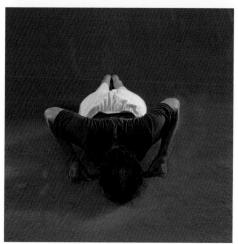

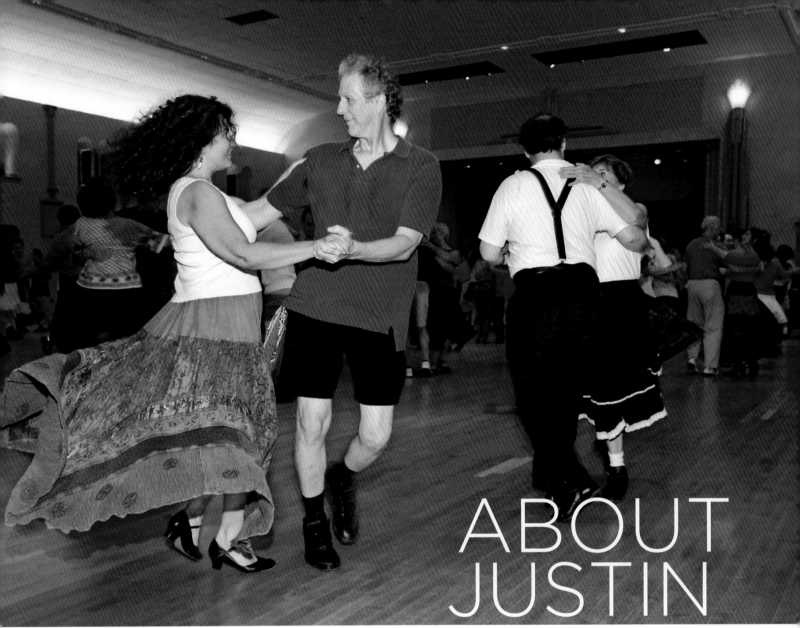

ABOUT JUSTIN

AGE	*56*
PROFESSION	*Fire alarm & security systems sales*
TYPE OF PRACTICE	*Hatha yoga, pranayama, meditation, contemplation*
LEVEL OF EXPERIENCE	*Advanced practitioner, teacher*
GREATEST BENEFIT OF THE PRACTICE TO JUSTIN	*Living in the natural flow of life.*
JUSTIN'S ADVICE TO OTHERS	*For beginners, start with not knowing. In yoga, as in life, there is no particular place to get to and no experience to achieve. Just practice and see what shows up. For experienced practitioners, identify those things about your practice of which you are certain and allow for the possibility that your next insight lies beyond that certainty.*

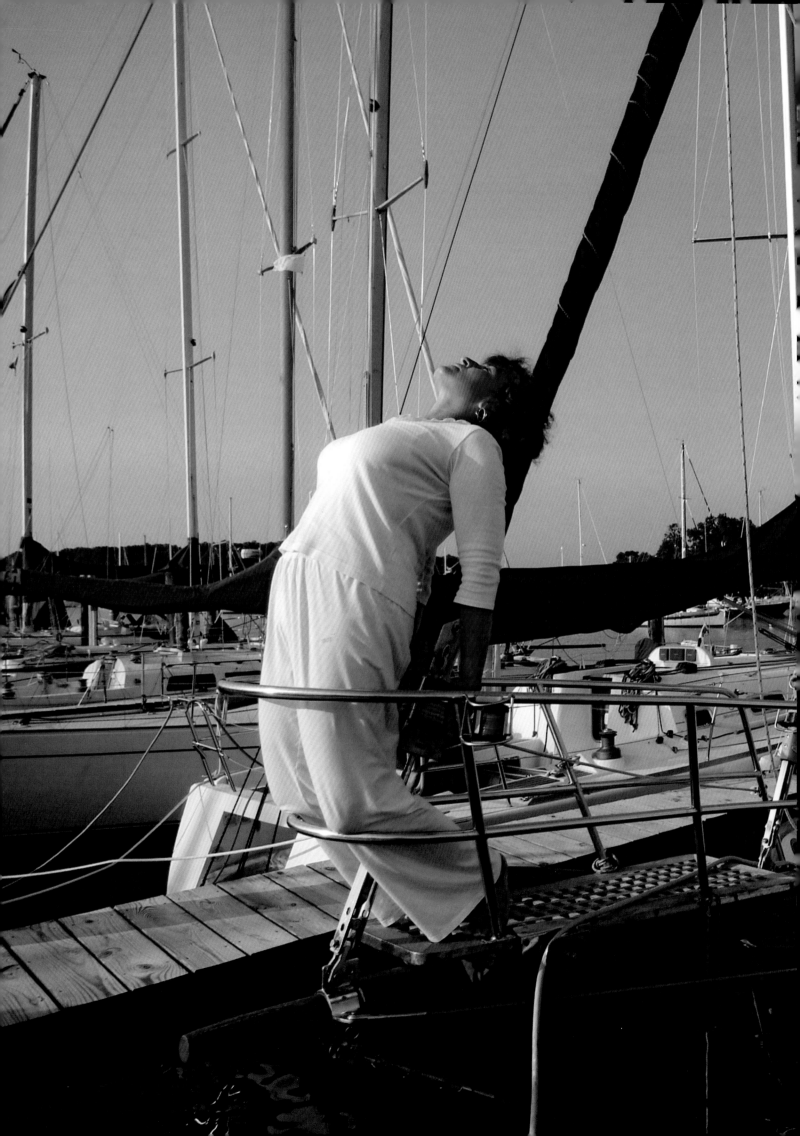

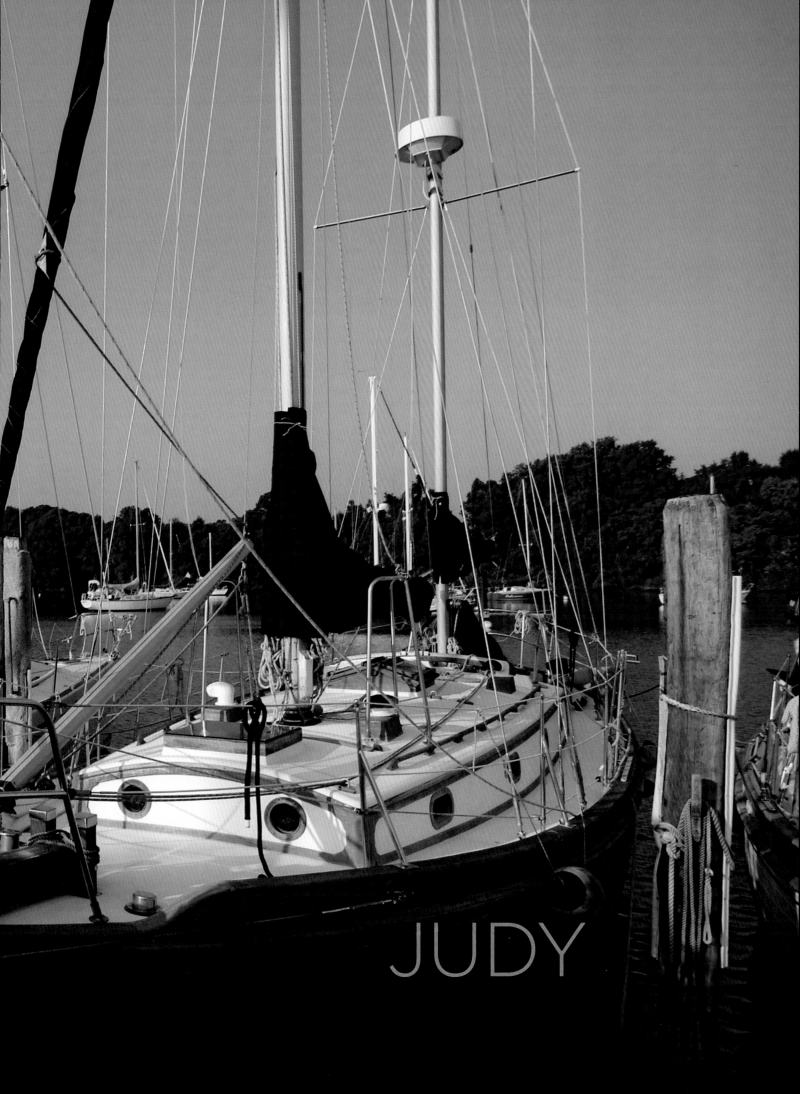

JUDY

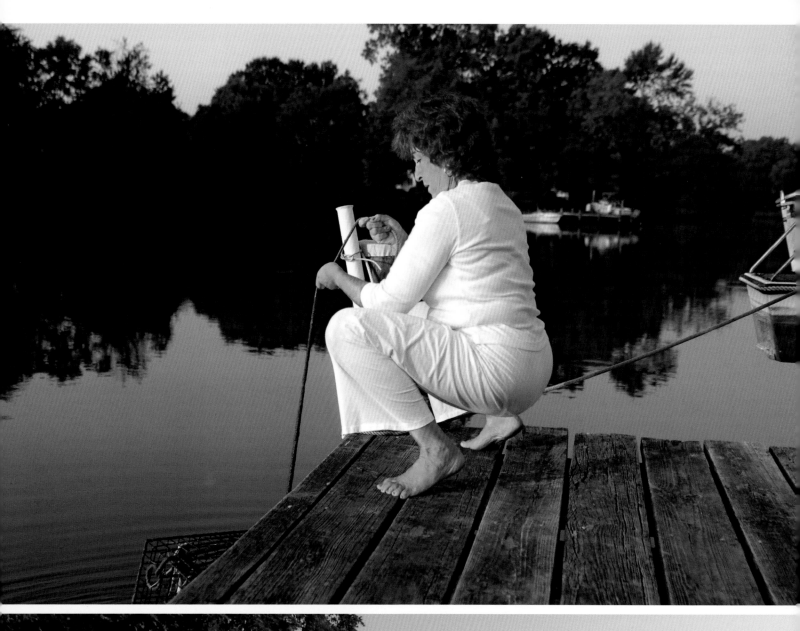
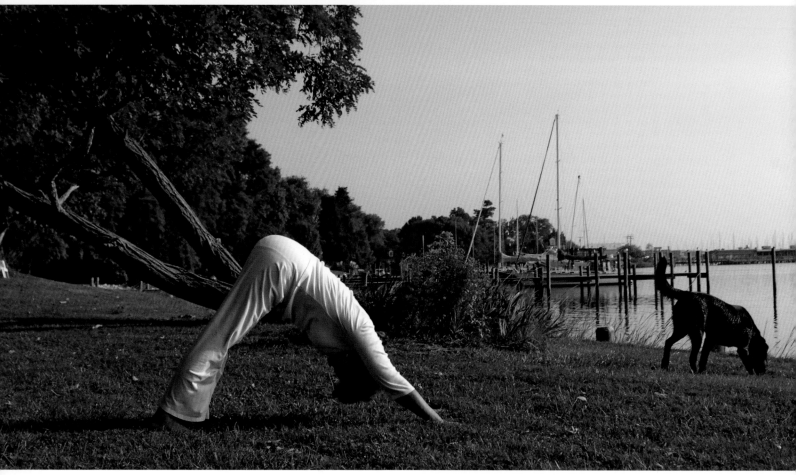

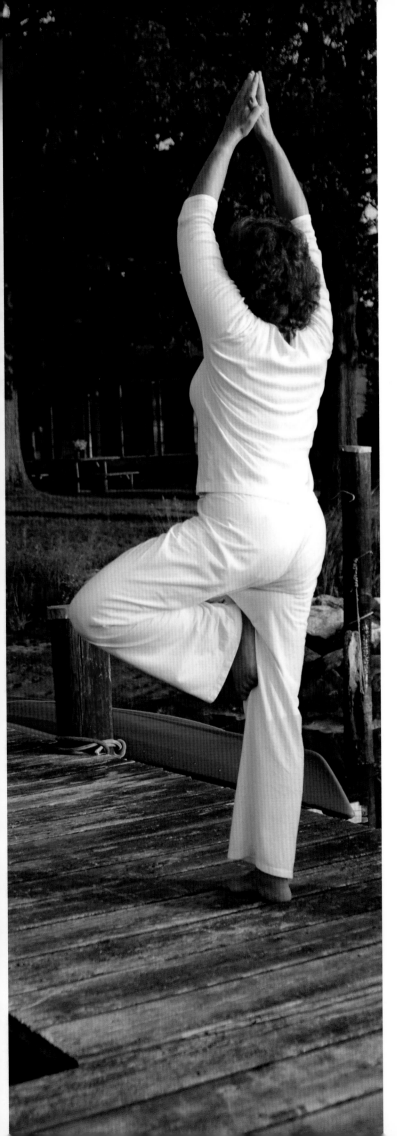

JUDY, A RETIRED OFFICE MANAGER AND RECREATIONAL SAILOR, challenges all comers to "join me in a sailboat race and see how I can move!" She adds that "not too many others my age can do what I can do and I owe it all to yoga."

Judy didn't always feel that way about yoga. Her first experience had been so negative that she thought she would never return. "Since my early twenties I had spent weeks at a time in bed unable to move because of back pain. A simple sneeze or sudden movement was enough to debilitate me." A friend suggested she try yoga. Everything else had failed so she enrolled in a class of about 25 students crammed into a cold basement. She got little effective instruction and soon gave up, "feeling as if I'd failed."

Months later, Judy says, "I desperately needed to feel better so I decided to give yoga one final try." Her first class was an instant success. She was impressed with the teacher's compassionate, careful approach and attention to detail. Ten years later, Judy continues to attend weekly classes. Yoga has become a staple in her life. "My awful back pain has disappeared," she says. More than that, "my energy level is very high. I am rarely tired and my yoga practice keeps me physically fit and able to race on sailboats, competing with people half my age."

It was natural for Judy to take her yoga practice into her sailing. "The biggest challenge is to get to my mat," she says. "It takes discipline, but once I realized I could practice anywhere the rest was easy." Judy enjoys creating new ways to unite her passion for being on the water with her love of yoga. She practices playfully at the water's edge while waiting for a big race or checking crab traps. Creative yoga provides Judy with a sense of liberation. "I feel like a butterfly emerging from my cocoon."

59

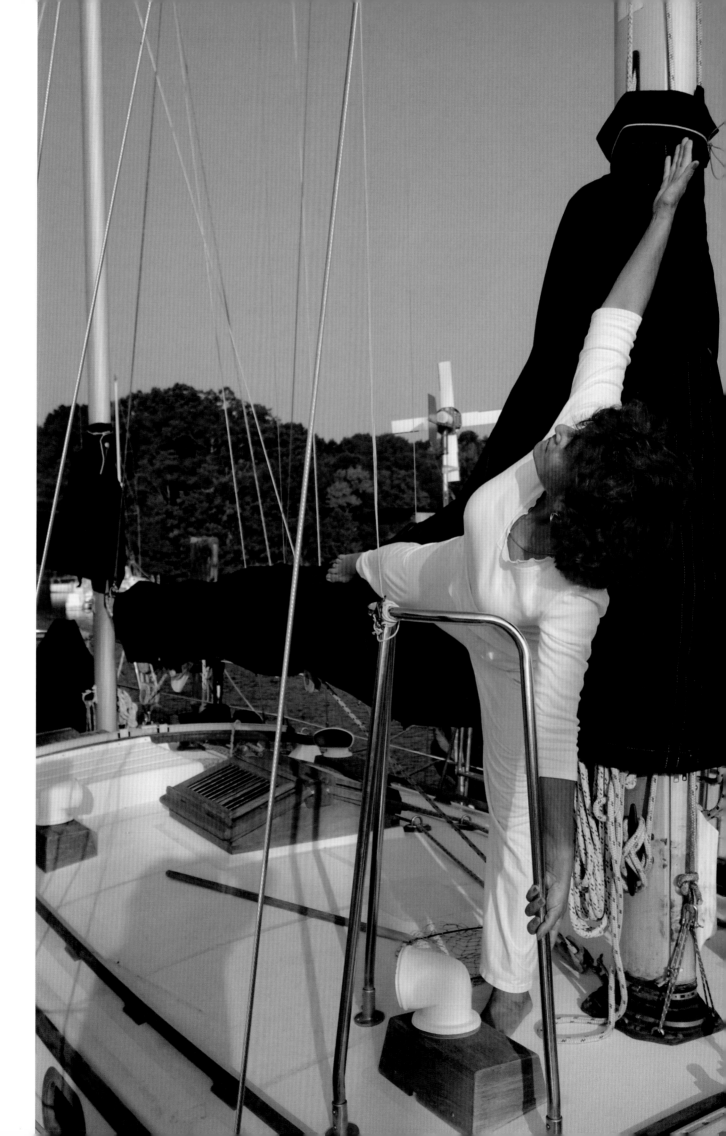

Free of nagging back pain, Judy has deepened into some of yoga's subtler benefits. She reports that "the ability to be still in mind and body" has been one of the greatest rewards of her practice. "Practicing yoga in any situation can be beneficial to everyone," she says, "whether you're driving in traffic, coping with health issues or dealing with grandchildren."

ABOUT JUDY

AGE	*64*
PROFESSION	*Retired office manager, full-time wife, mother & grandmother*
TYPE OF PRACTICE	*Hatha Yoga*
LEVEL OF EXPERIENCE	*10 years*
GREATEST BENEFIT OF THE PRACTICE TO JUDY	*Total relief from back pain, high energy, the ability to be still in body and mind.*
JUDY'S ADVICE TO OTHERS	*No matter what your age or physical condition, you can improve your life with yoga. Keep looking until you find the right teacher and then enjoy!*

HUY

"I WAS LOOKING FOR INSPIRATION," SAYS HUY, a high-energy 34-year-old martial artist and admitted "peak performance junkie." The chief financial officer of a non-profit organization, Huy had spent his 20s immersed in business studies, break-dancing, high-technology marketing, Tae Kwon Do and Kung Fu.

Huy abandoned the pursuit of material success in favor of an "authentic life" choosing advanced Kung Fu study over a master's degree in business administration. It was an "unconventional" choice, he says, but it set him on his life-long path of self-discovery. He married and had children, and he continued to seek ways to feel centered and grounded while bolstering his drive for adventure and achievement.

Then he found a yoga teacher who "integrated our physical experience with our mental and emotional states," Huy says. She'd confront her students with statements such as "imagine that you have five minutes to live and you have no choice but to maintain this pose. How does that influence your intention or your experience?"

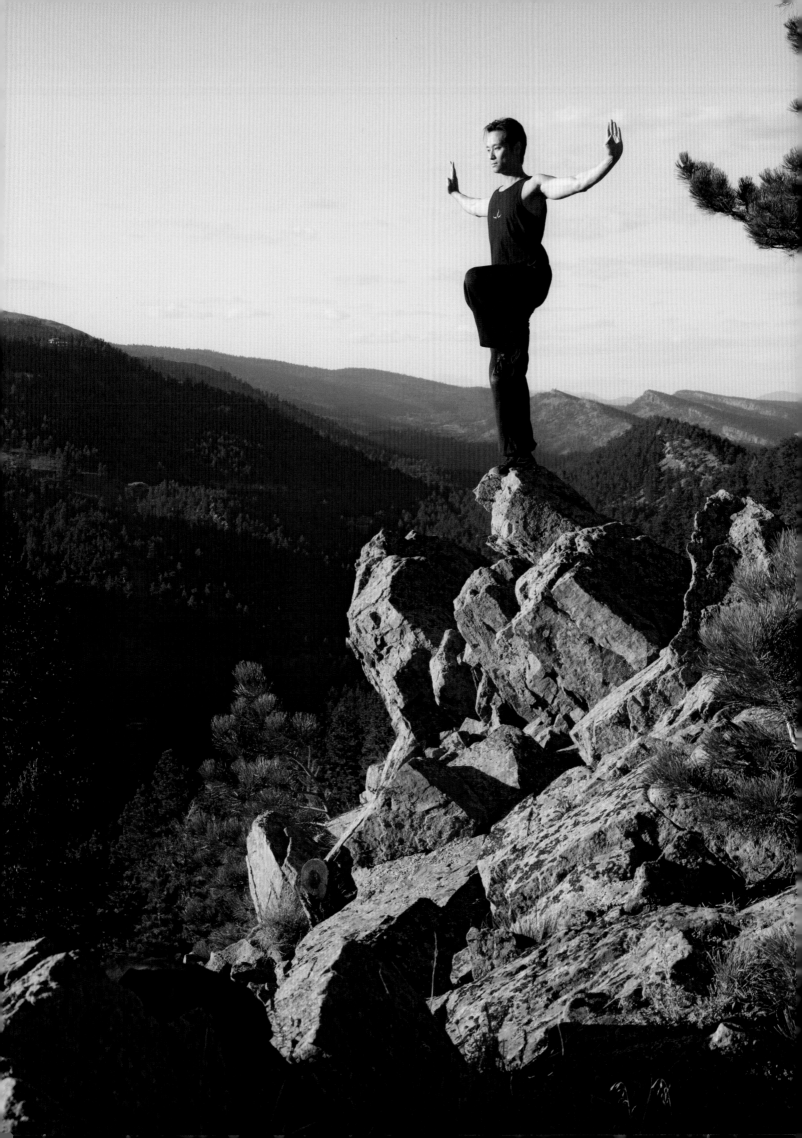

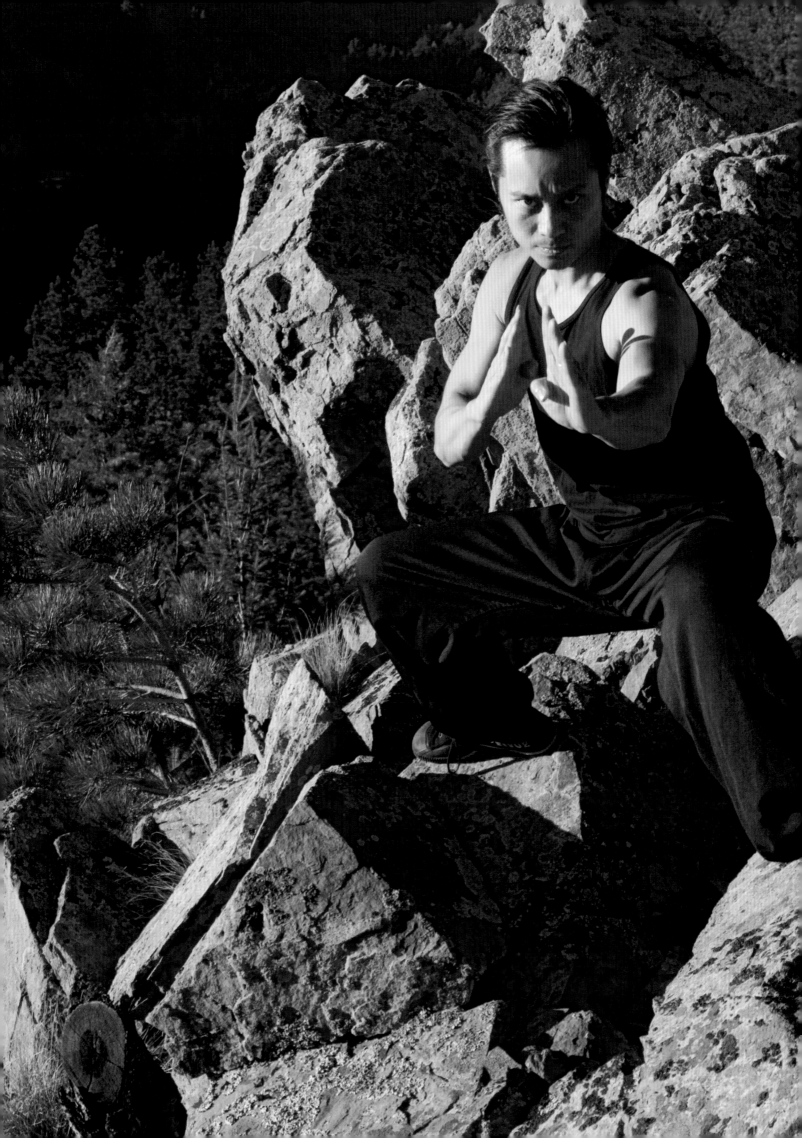

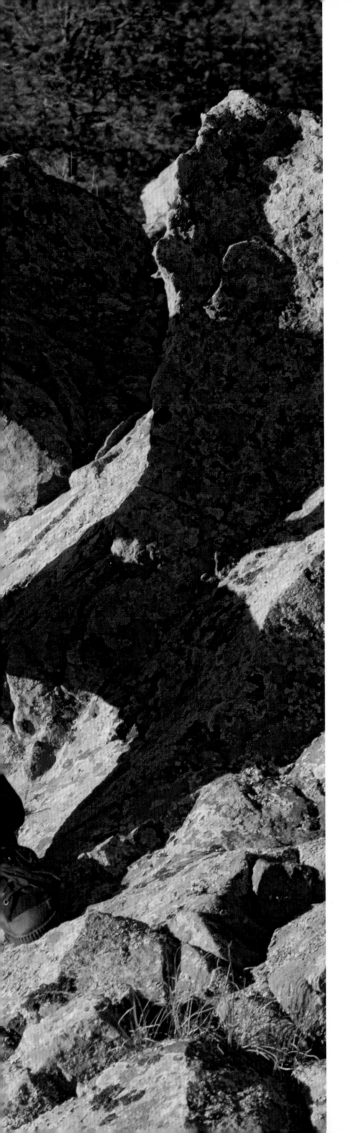

"Yoga has taught me that nothing has to change physically during times of challenge but if you shift your focus and alter your attitude you become free of negative experience," he says. "Of course, learning to apply this in yoga is the same thing as learning to apply it in life." Huy successfully brings this mindset to all aspects of his life. His yoga practice has become "an expression of who I am." The principles of yoga continue to inspire him to excel in all areas of his life, especially when he feels stretched to his limit at work, at home and on the mat.

"The art of life and the art of yoga are the same," says Huy, "It's all about what you do with the experience of being at your edge."

ABOUT HUY

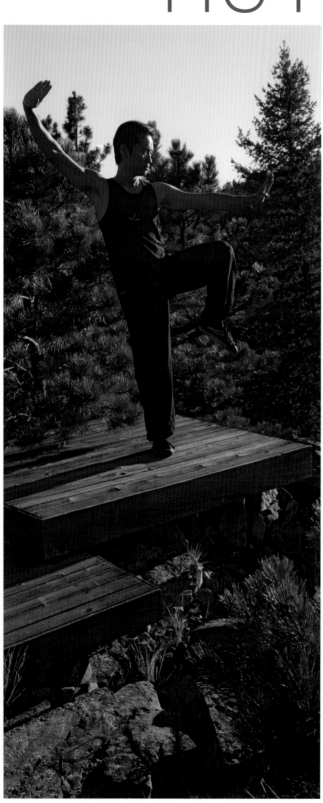

AGE	*34*
PROFESSION	*Chief Financial Officer*
TYPE OF PRACTICE	*Hatha Yoga*
LEVEL OF EXPERIENCE	*6 years*
GREATEST BENEFIT OF THE PRACTICE TO HUY	*The integrative quality; simultaneously bringing focus to internal and external experience*
HUY'S ADVICE TO OTHERS	*See yoga as a tool for learning to be free in the midst of challenge. When you reach your edge, stay there and manage your thoughts and emotions as a way to release yourself from negative mental habits.*

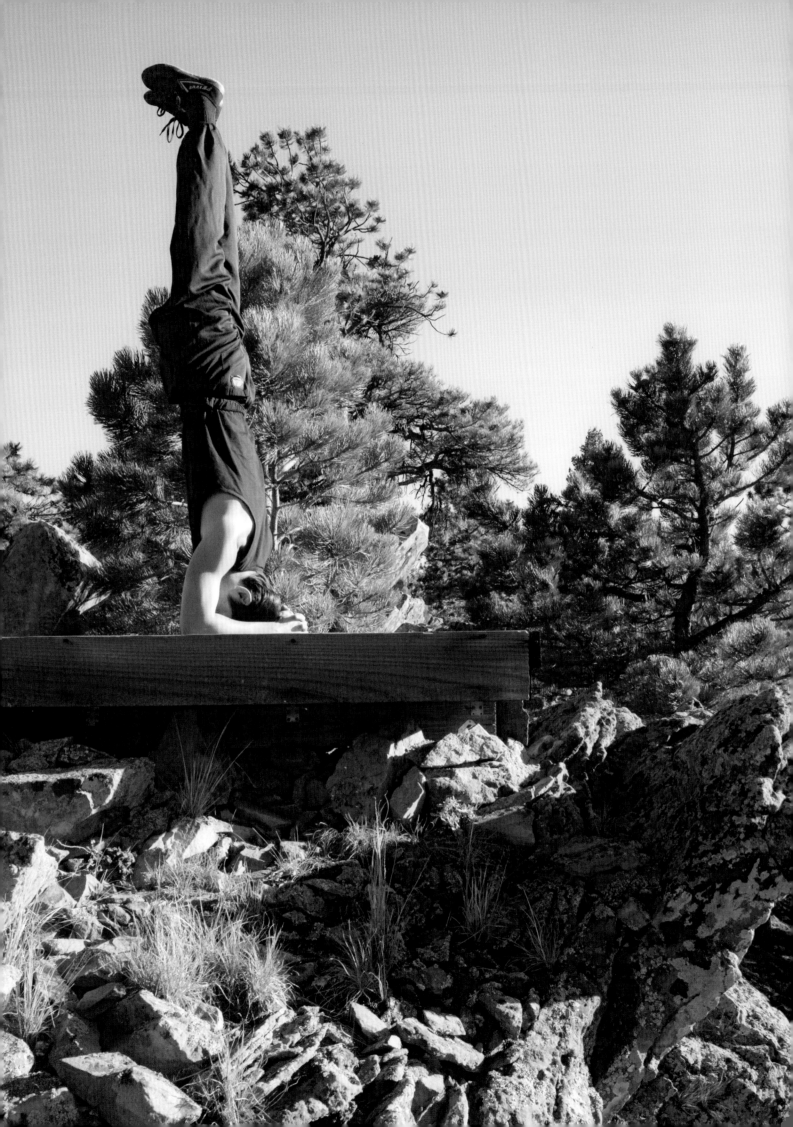

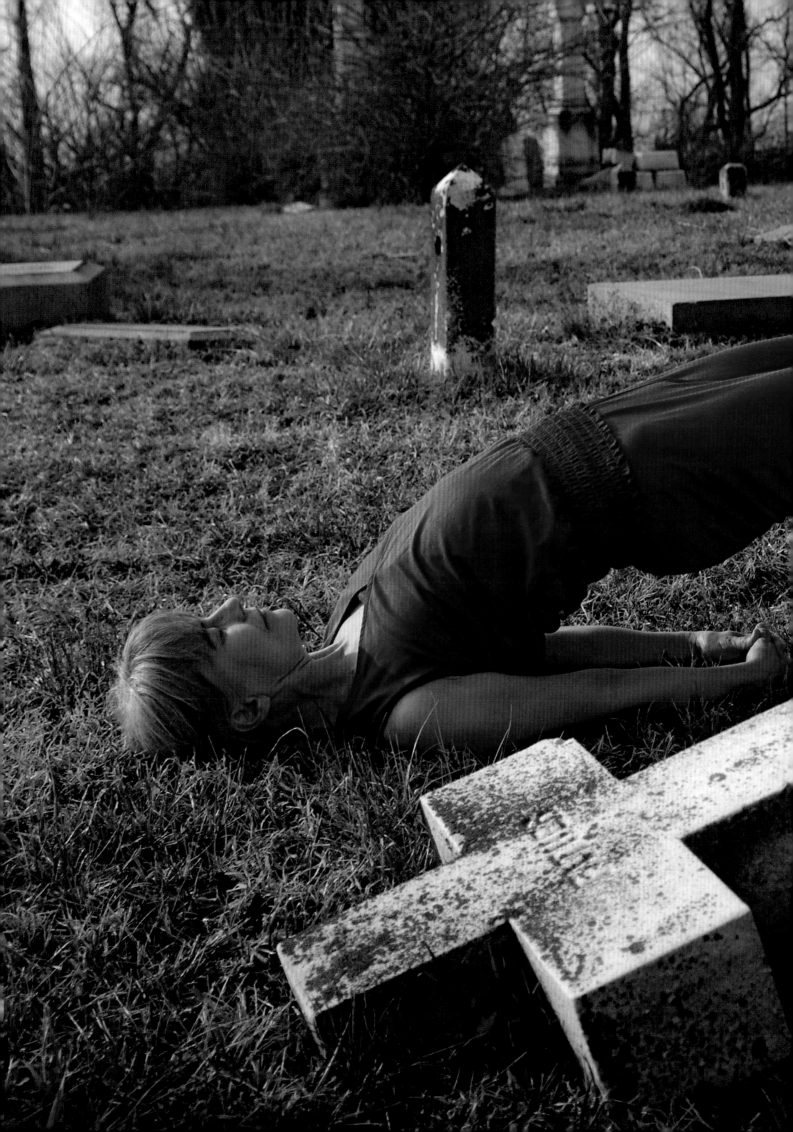

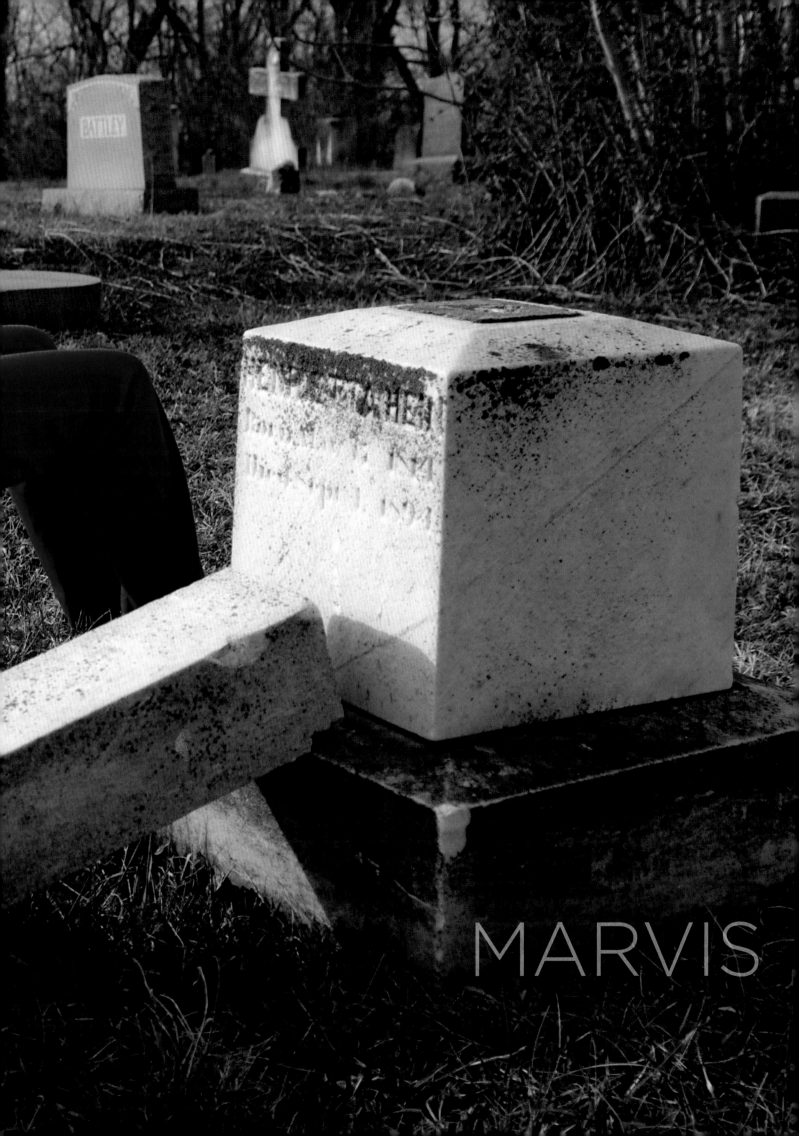

MARVIS

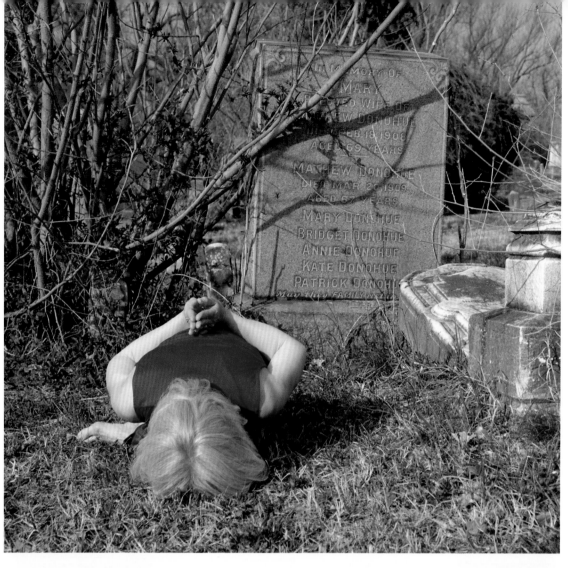

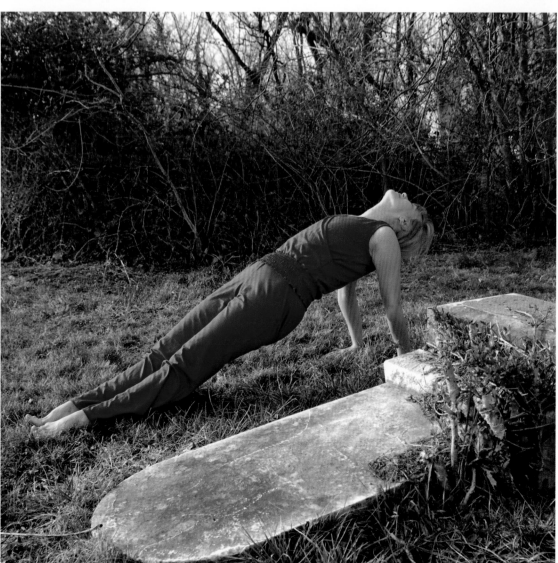

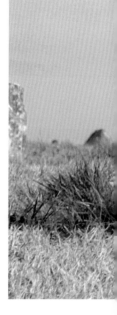

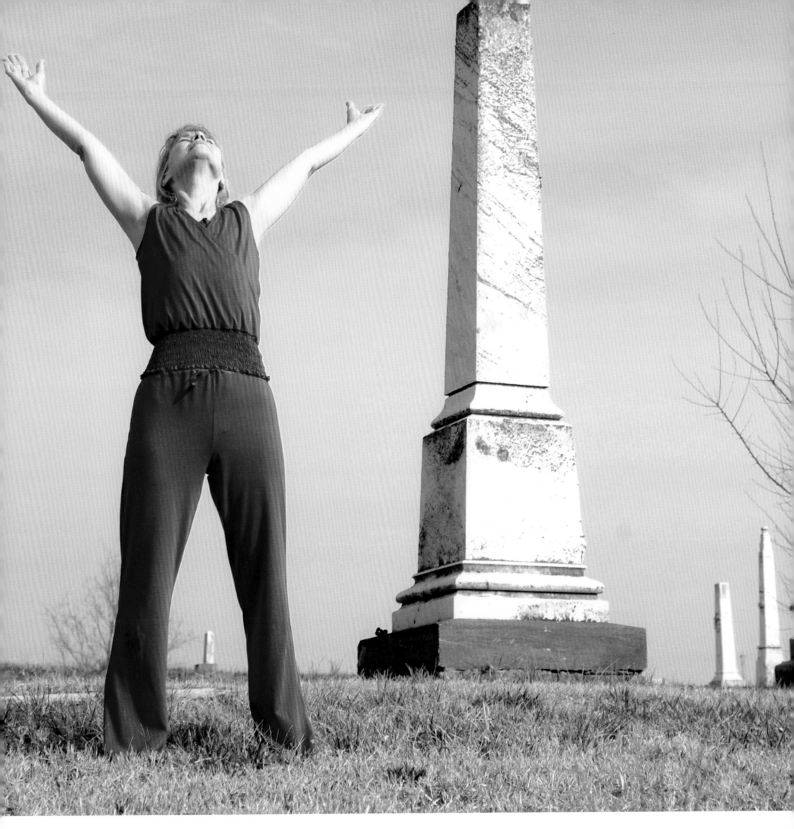

MARVIS IS A POET ... AND A
BREAST CANCER SURVIVOR.
At age 66 she "lives life wide awake" and her
daily hatha yoga practice ensures that her
senses are open and receptive. She sees the
ordinary in extraordinary ways: the "yellow
eyed wolf moon" casting "cold, dark shadows
in the primeval forest." She knows, at first
hand, the fragility of life and the certainty of
impermanence and she relies on her yoga
practice to "deepen my appreciation of the
varied opportunities presented anew each day."

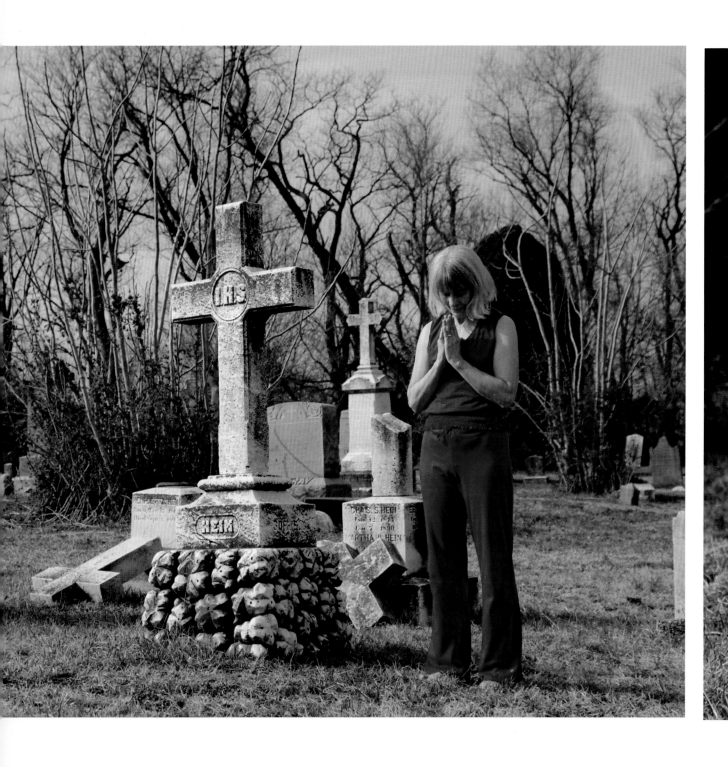

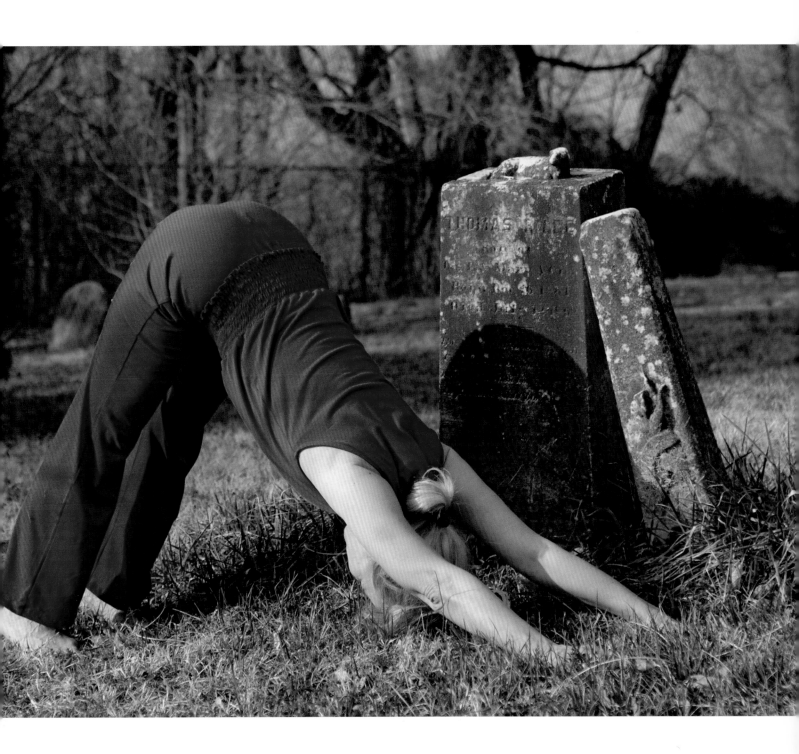

IN MARVIS' WORDS:

The abandoned cemetery hovers beside passersby, unnoticed; the epitome of what is just
out of sight, out of mind. It defines impermanence, a stark reminder of the unfolding cycle as
the universe breathes us into being, over and over. It speaks silently of how much more we
are than the boundaries of our bodies and our present names.

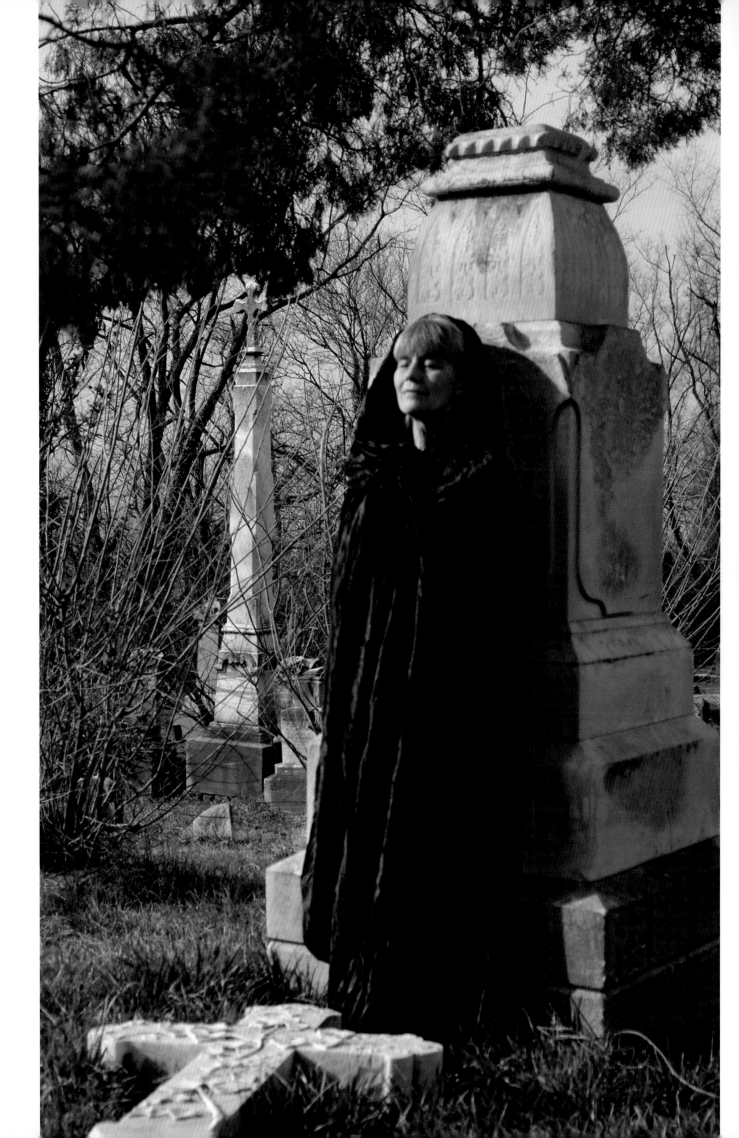

The wind, the rain,
Were never
Fooled

Illusions
Set in stone

Remnants
Of identities,
Erased

Captured time,
Released

Crumbled ruins
Sacred space

Faint traces
Of ancient memories

Yoga, to me, is the holding of opposites. A yoga practice embodies discipline and freedom, structure and spontaneity, sensory messages from the body and voices of the mind. It is the sacred act of marrying the present moment with timelessness. The reward is the bliss of finding the essence of a pose, releasing all effort and being held by breath alone. Yoga is my path to being open to the challenges and adventures of passing through the thresholds that open before me on the journey I call my life.

ABOUT MARVIS

AGE *66*

PROFESSION *Real Estate Office Manager*

TYPE OF PRACTICE *Hatha Yoga*

LEVEL OF EXPERIENCE *13 years daily practice*

GREATEST BENEFIT OF THE PRACTICE TO MARVIS *Gaining the strength and flexibility to take on the challenges and opportunities of life and exploring what lies beneath.*

MARVIS' ADVICE TO OTHERS *Let your yoga be an expression of your life. Let your yoga be a river, flowing around obstacles, cutting through time, remembering that rainbows are created from plunging over falls and the journey is the destination.*

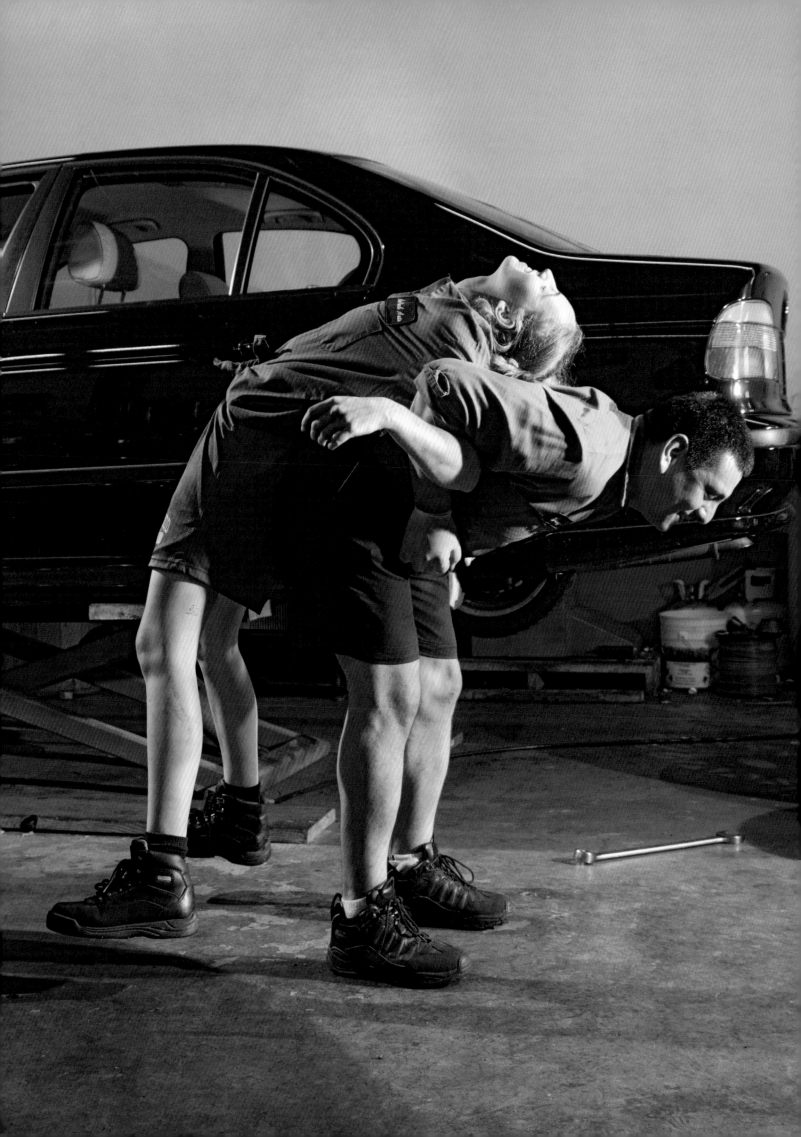

MANNY, 44, OWNS AND RUNS A garage that specializes in maintaining and repairing high-performance vehicles. Yoga wasn't one of Manny's tools before Kate began to work for him as a part-time mechanic. And when Kate first tried to get Manny to join her in "yoga breaks" he wasn't particularly interested.

"Working on cars can be so frustrating at times that it makes me want to scream," Kate says. So she channeled her frustration into inventing new yoga positions. "My body gets a good release, I forget that I'm irritated, and I get the boost I need to go back to wrestling with screws that refuse to turn and heavy engine parts that don't want to fit together."

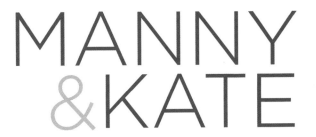

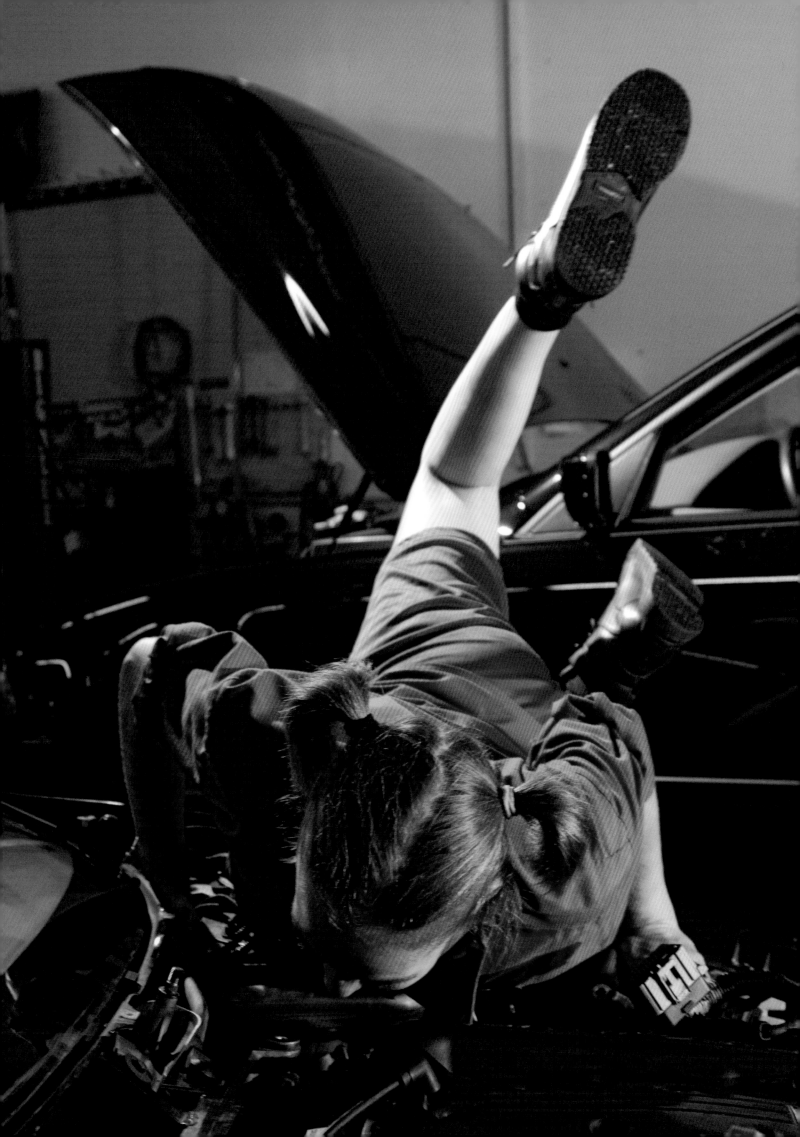

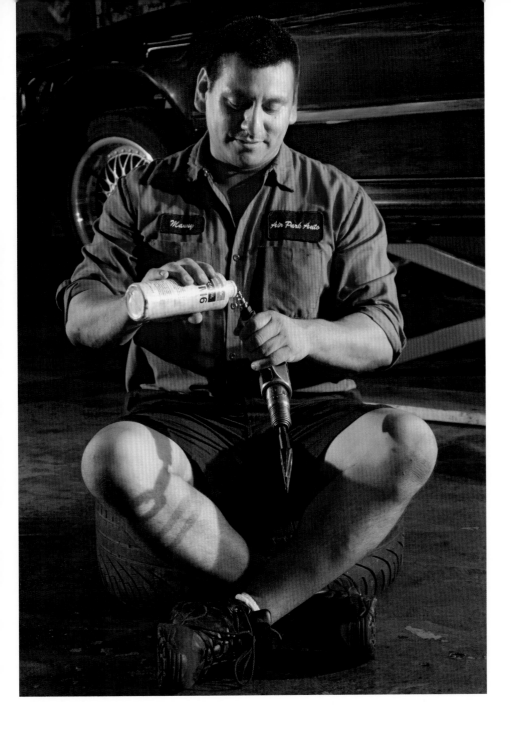

One day, Kate convinced Manny to "take a yoga break instead of a coffee break." His first discovery was that it eased his chronic back pain. "I feel great and now I'm hooked!" he says. These days he enjoys creating his own yoga at work. " I never imagined I'd be able to stretch this far. When I let my body weight go into a stretch, the release is amazing. Best of all ... I'm pain free!"

Manny also found that yoga helped him cope with the stress of dealing with clients with high expectations and little tolerance for mistakes and delays. "Disappointed customers can be pretty cranky," but yoga helps him "take it all in stride," Manny says.

Manny and Kate now do yoga workouts together. "I can't believe how much fun it is," says Manny. Yoga "lifts the spirits of everyone who comes into the shop," Kate says. "It's infectious. When we're more relaxed and happy, our customers are too."

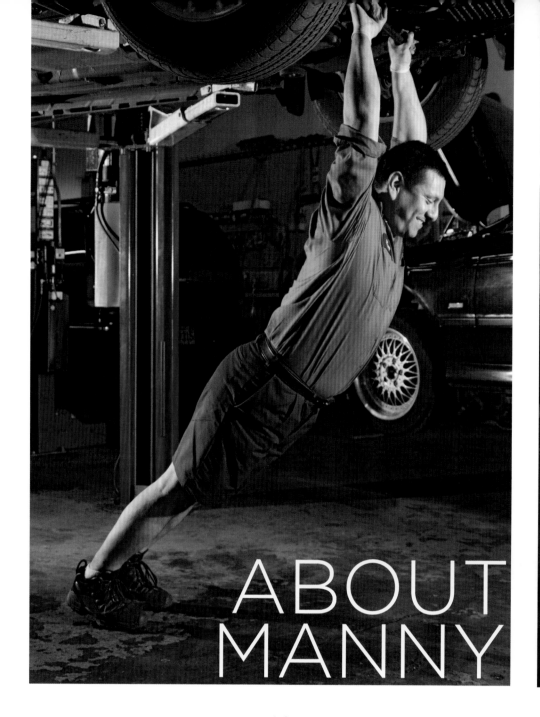

ABOUT MANNY

AGE	*44*
PROFESSION	*Entreprenuer; master mechanic*
TYPE OF PRACTICE	*Spontaneous, creative hatha yoga*
LEVEL OF EXPERIENCE	*Complete beginner*
GREATEST BENEFIT OF THE PRACTICE TO MANNY	*Self-awareness, body awareness*
MANNY'S ADVICE TO OTHERS	*Let go of preconceived notions. Approach yoga with a totally open mind.*

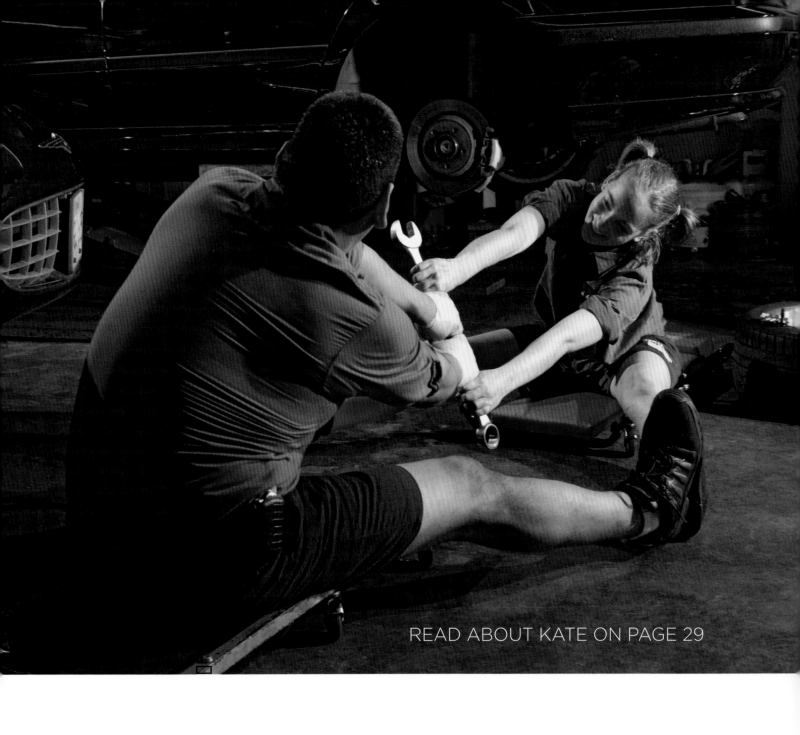

READ ABOUT KATE ON PAGE 29

AMY MET KEVIN EIGHT YEARS AGO while interviewing potential housemates. She liked everything about him and instantly turned him down, explaining that she was far too attracted to him to be comfortable sharing a house. Kevin smiled broadly and asked Amy out to dinner. The rest, as they say, is history ... and her story ... and their story.

Amy, a 42 year-old massage therapist had been practicing yoga for 15 years as an antidote to the "noise and pace" of urban life. As an organic gardener, reared in the quiet hills of California, Amy felt that her move to the east coast plunged her into sensory overload. She observed the benefits of yoga while sharing a house with two yoga teachers. Convinced to give it a try, Amy quickly learned to use "breathing techniques as stress busters and energy movers." Her practice has morphed over the years from primarily being a stress management tool to providing her with "increased strength and flexibility."

Kevin, age 46, is now Amy's only housemate and yoga partner. An aerospace engineer and an enthusiastic black-belt martial artist, Kevin had yoga nowhere on his radar screen until he met Amy. His admiration for her "quiet wisdom" and "strong, flexible body" moved him to join her. At first, it was a new and interesting way to spend time with Amy. He now comes to his mat every other day and "lives the principles of yoga every day."

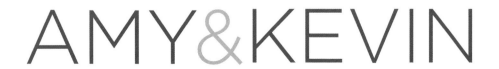

AMY&KEVIN

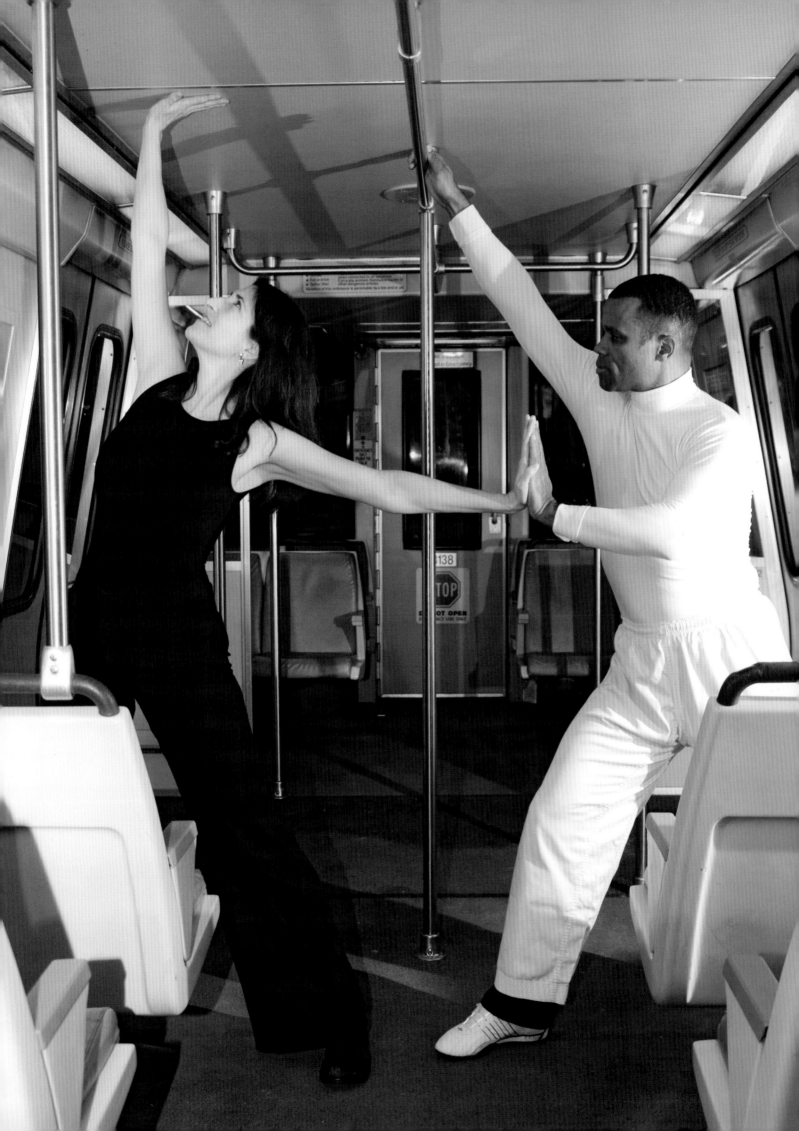

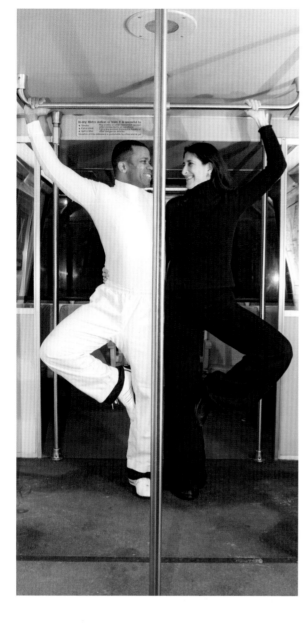

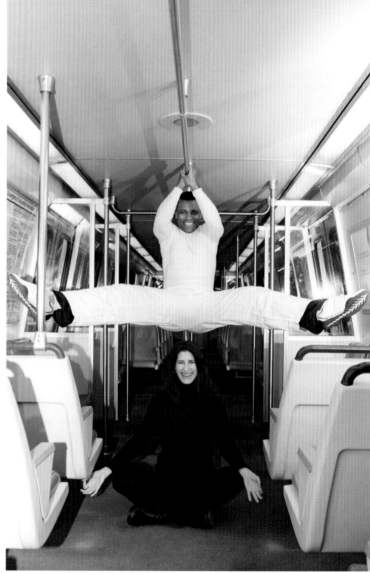

Kevin and Amy are opposites in many ways. He is fiercely goal directed. She is deeply process oriented. He loves meat. She's a vegetarian. He kicks and punches for recreation. She plants flowers and vegetables. They appreciate the yin and yang of their relationship.

They decided to try their yoga on a Washington, D.C. Metro train as a way of expressing their love of paradox. They both liked the idea of bringing their relaxed, relational yoga practice to the impersonal, stressful environment of a rushing commuter train. "I love the rush of life," says Kevin, "but I also love relaxing and relating."

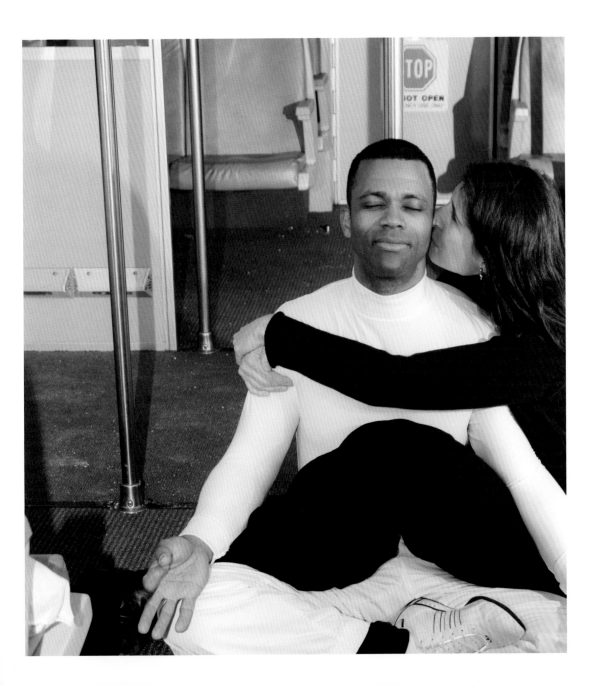

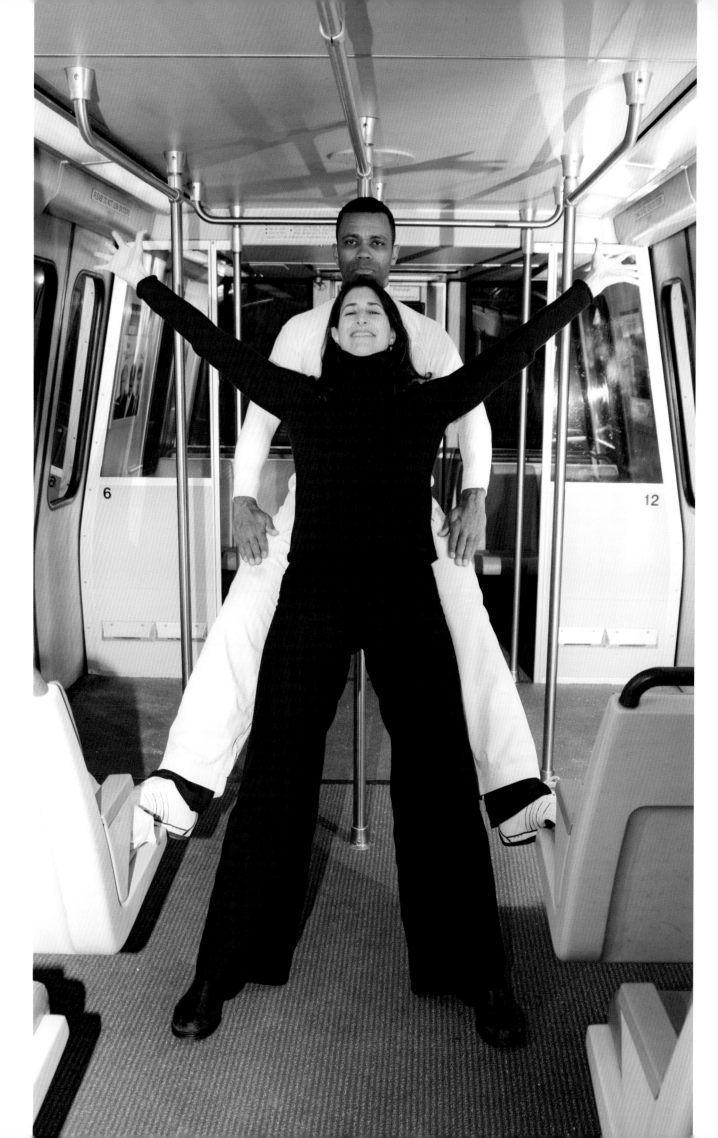

ABOUT AMY

AGE	*42*
PROFESSION	*Massage therapist*
TYPE OF PRACTICE	*Eclectic*
LEVEL OF EXPERIENCE	*15 years, but who's counting?*
GREATEST BENEFIT OF THE PRACTICE TO AMY	*Peace of mind and physical strength and flexibility.*
AMY'S ADVICE	*The benefits are so many and it feels so good. Why would you not do yoga? It's important to find the right type of yoga for you at any given time (and there are lots!) If you're just starting, find a really good teacher so that you get a positive introduction to the practice you choose.*

ABOUT KEVIN

AGE	*46*
PROFESSION	*Aerospace engineer/aviation meteorologist*
TYPE OF PRACTICE	*Eclectic*
LEVEL OF EXPERIENCE	*Six months*
GREATEST BENEFIT OF THE PRACTICE TO KEVIN	*Physical, psychological, and spiritual awareness, and agility.*
KEVIN'S ADVICE	*Your yoga practice will become an expression of how valuable a fully developed 'you' can be to a developing relationship and to your world.*

SHARON, AGE 36, IS A FULL-TIME MOTHER AND PART-TIME CERTIFIED YOGA INSTRUCTOR. "I practice my yoga constantly, on and off the mat," she says. She relies on her yoga practice to keep her calm, flexible, and strong while responding to the unceasing demands of motherhood. "My children challenge me to temper my emotions and to cultivate compassion," she says.

With two young children at home and pregnant with her third, Sharon says her days are filled with opportunities to creatively put her yoga to work. Whether it's finding the patience to encourage her son through his piano practice or settling in for story time with her daughter, Sharon mindfully applies yoga's physical alignment principles. "I'm stronger and have fewer aches and pains," she says. Beyond the physical benefits, Sharon is better able to deal with the inevitable everyday upsets of motherhood. Yoga helps her to shift her perspective "and see myself from the point of view of Universal Presence."

Pregnancy taxes the mind and body in countless ways and Sharon takes on the challenge with ease. Prenatal yoga helps to create a positive and nourishing intrauterine environment and prepares her and her unborn baby for the most profound journey of their shared existence.

SHARON

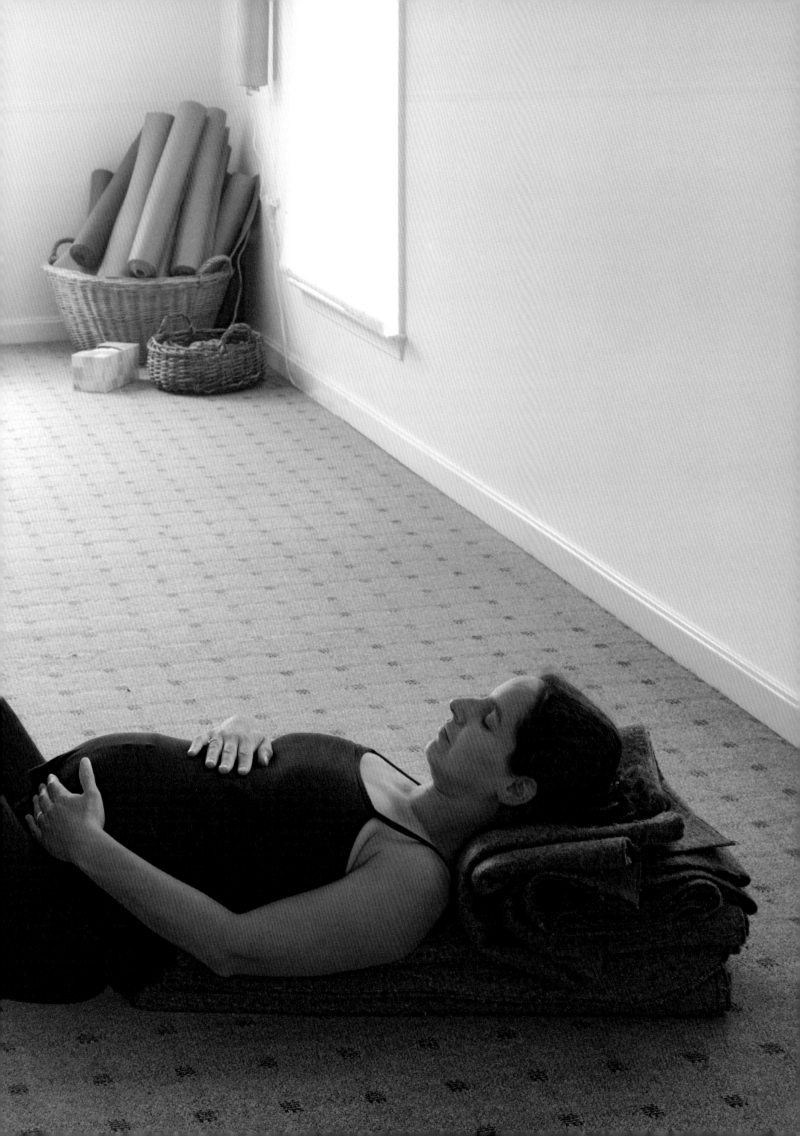

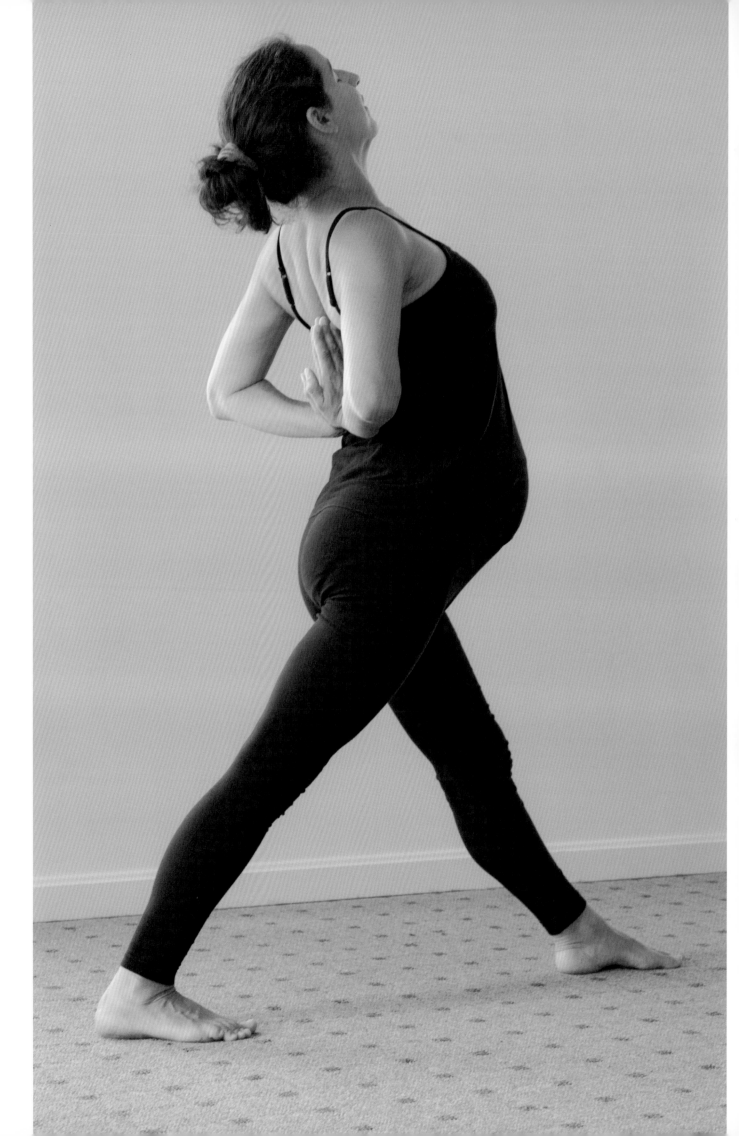

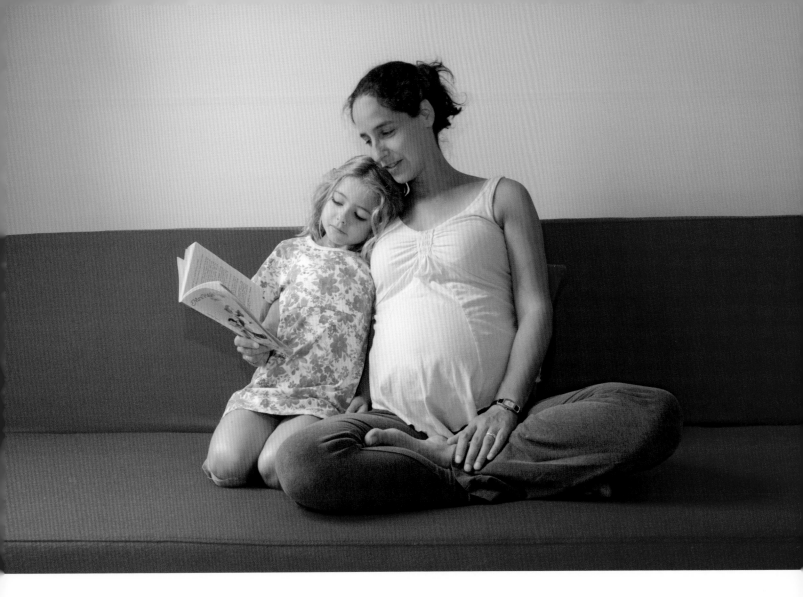

Sharon's prenatal practice not only prepares her body for the rigors of labor and delivery, "It reminds me that I am connected to something beyond myself and that my true nature is bliss."

As a certified Anusara™ Yoga teacher, she reaps the rewards of yoga's unifying influence. "I came to yoga looking for a physical discipline to help me release nervous tension. The benefits I've enjoyed go far beyond that," she says. "I never feel isolated" —and neither does anyone who knows her. The warmth of Sharon's spirit sparks a light in everyone she meets.

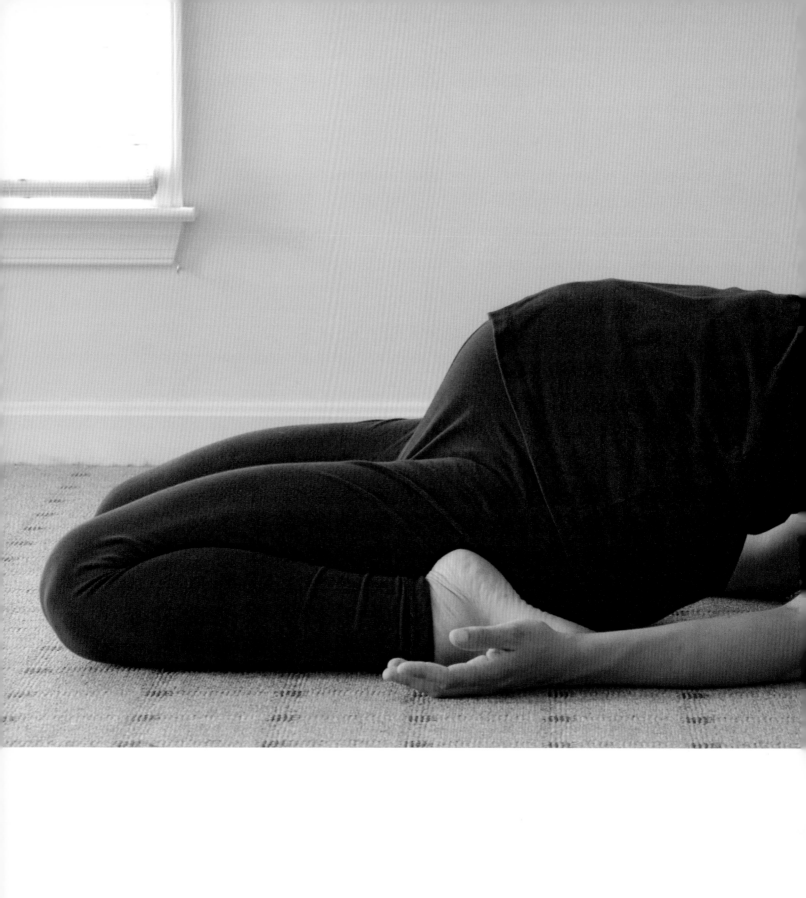

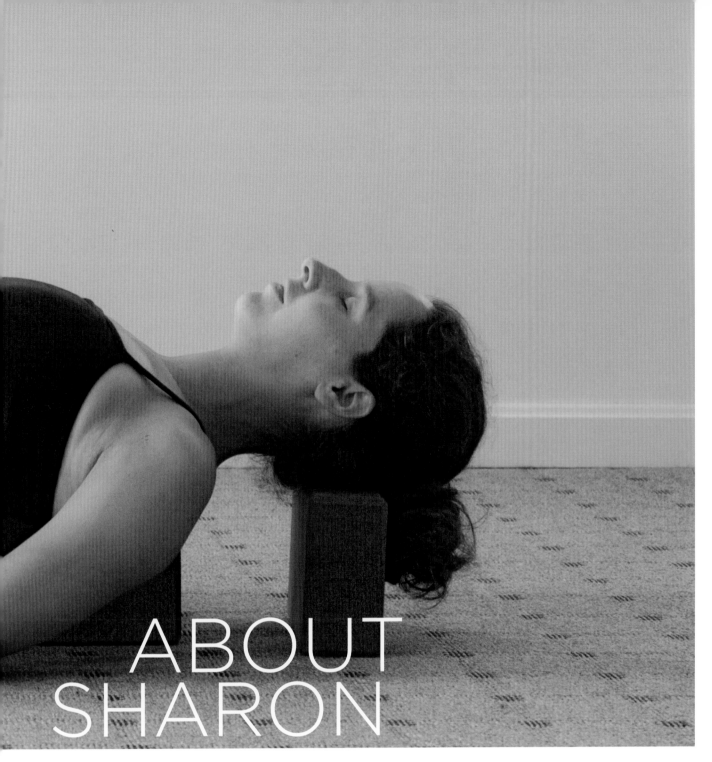

ABOUT SHARON

AGE	*36*
PROFESSION	*Full-time mother, part-time yoga instructor*
TYPE OF PRACTICE	*Anusara™/mindful flow*
LEVEL OF EXPERIENCE	*10 years*
GREATEST BENEFIT OF THE PRACTICE TO SHARON	*Belonging to a community, strength & flexibility, fewer aches and pains, improved patience, and overall well being.*
SHARON'S ADVICE TO OTHERS	*When you know and help your self through yoga, you recognize your own divine nature and can therefore recognize that same essence in all beings.*

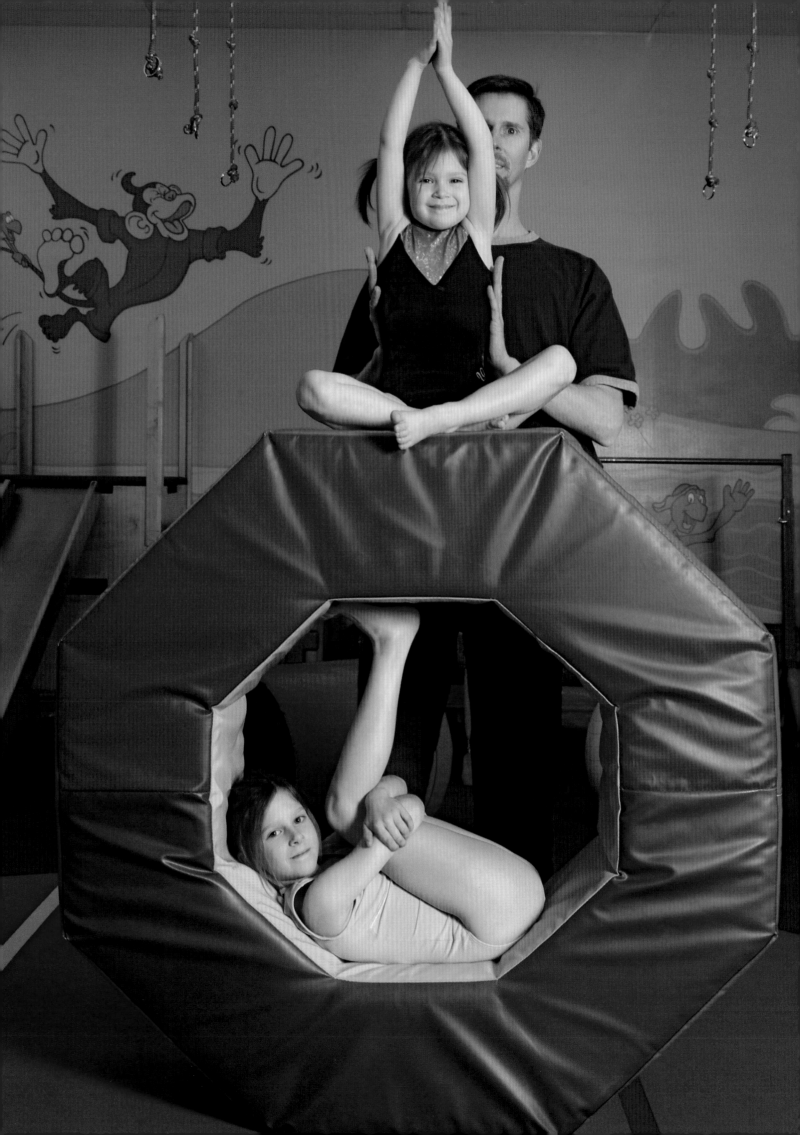

"I HAD BEEN PUTTING IN 11-HOUR WORKDAYS and traveling 3 to 5 days a week by the time my second daughter was born. The job of parenting had fallen completely to my wife and I began to feel like a weekend visitor in my own home."

A manager at an information technology firm, Alan worked his way to professional success and financial security, believing that being the provider meant sacrificing time with his wife, his children and himself. At age 40, longing to participate in the life of his family, he felt stressed, spiritually drained, adrift.

Then, approaching personal burnout and suffering from chronic back pain, Alan experimented with a yoga class.

"It was like coming home. I learned to relax and feel comfortable in stillness" in the supportive environment of the yoga studio where he felt an easy kinship with other students along with a trust that he wasn't being judged or compared with anyone. Alan says. "I was able to let go of my competitive nature and feel the joy of just being. My body felt better, my mind cleared, and I reconnected with a spiritual aspect of myself that had been lying dormant since college."

Alan, raised a Catholic, had been attracted to Eastern philosophy and spiritual practices since his college days, and was particularly drawn to Buddhism, with its emphasis on transcending ego to

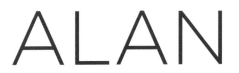

ALAN

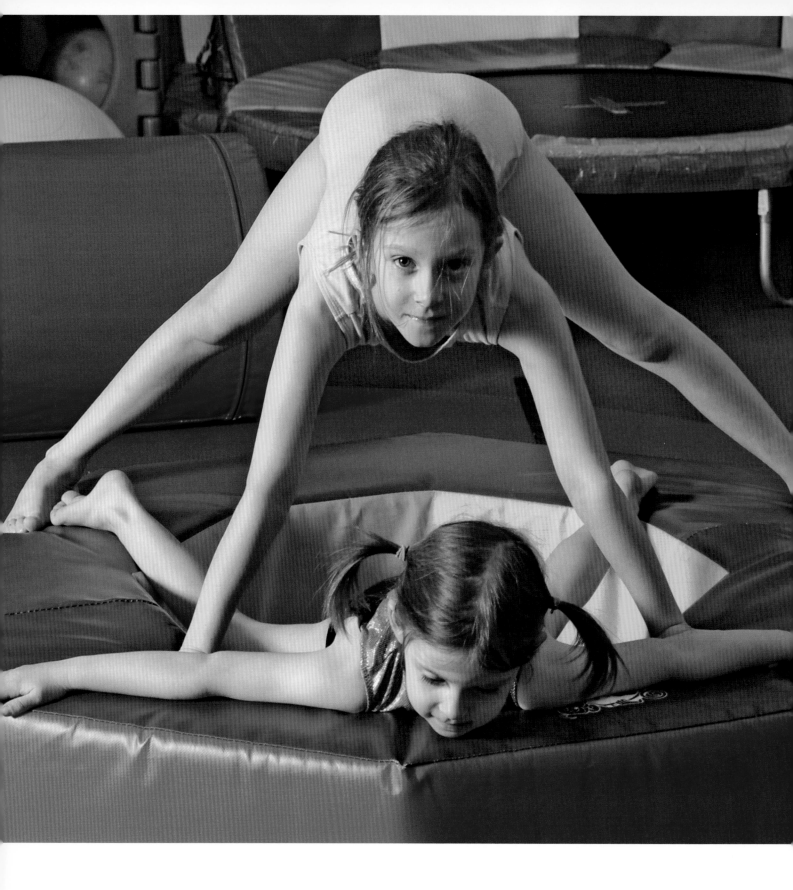

unite with the Divine. He and his wife, also raised Catholic, included a passage from the Baghavad Gita in their wedding readings, finding common ground between Christian teachings and Hindu principles.

As Alan turned his energy toward supporting his family he gradually began to realize that he'd lost touch with his Eastern spirituality. It troubled him and

he felt moved to find a way to reintroduce Eastern values into his life.

"Yoga means union," explains Alan, adding that it is his heartfelt intention to integrate his dearly held Eastern principles with the Christian values embraced by his family. "Yoga acts as a bridge," he says, "I can bring my philosophy into my family life in a gentle,

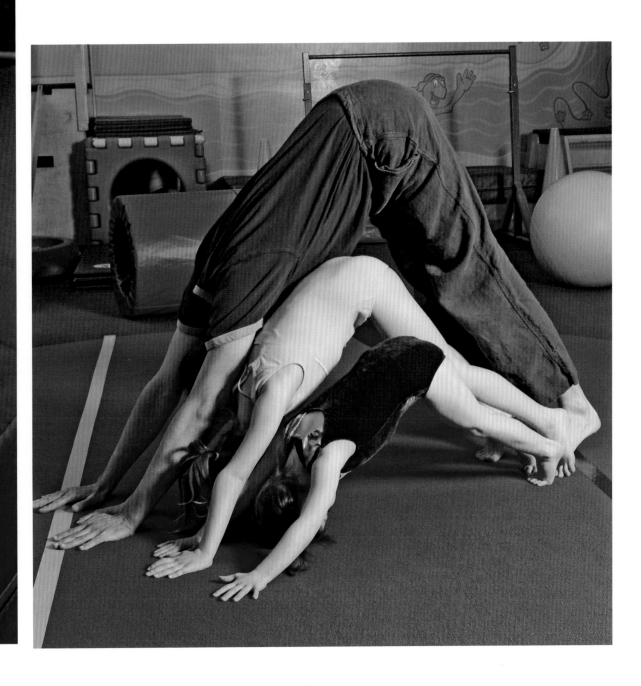

non-intrusive way. I can show the girls through example, that it's possible to be inclusive and spiritually multi-faceted without losing your fundamental beliefs."

Alan credits yoga for rejuvenating his values of spiritual generosity, compassion, non-harming and respect for all sentient beings. He has committed himself to maintaining a strong presence in the family, living moment-by-moment as a positive role model.

"Yoga has a balancing effect in my life. It provides a kind of leveling that keeps me from getting wrapped up in my own anxious worries. I am better able to connect in a caring way with others, especially my daughters."

A football watching, beer-drinking dad,

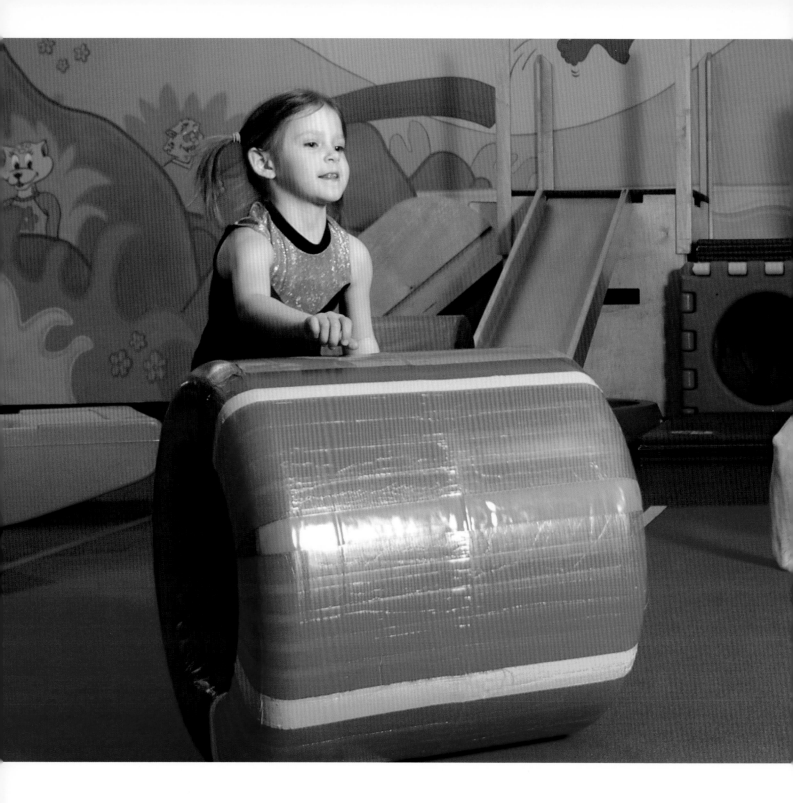

Alan has found that he enjoys taking a high-spirited yoga break with his girls every now and then. "I don't play with dolls," Alan explains with a lighthearted smile, so he likes to be able to pull yoga out of the toy box. "Pretend to be a tree. What sort of mountain do you want to be? Let's make up some poses of our own!" Alan's daughters have "taken my yoga to the next level!"

He says, "It's in keeping with so many of the great stories of spiritual growth. The student becomes the teacher. The child is the parent of the man. My girls have taught me to bring joy, exuberance and imagination to my practice!" He reports that yoga has made him a better person and a better father, adding, "It was my yoga, but now it's our yoga."

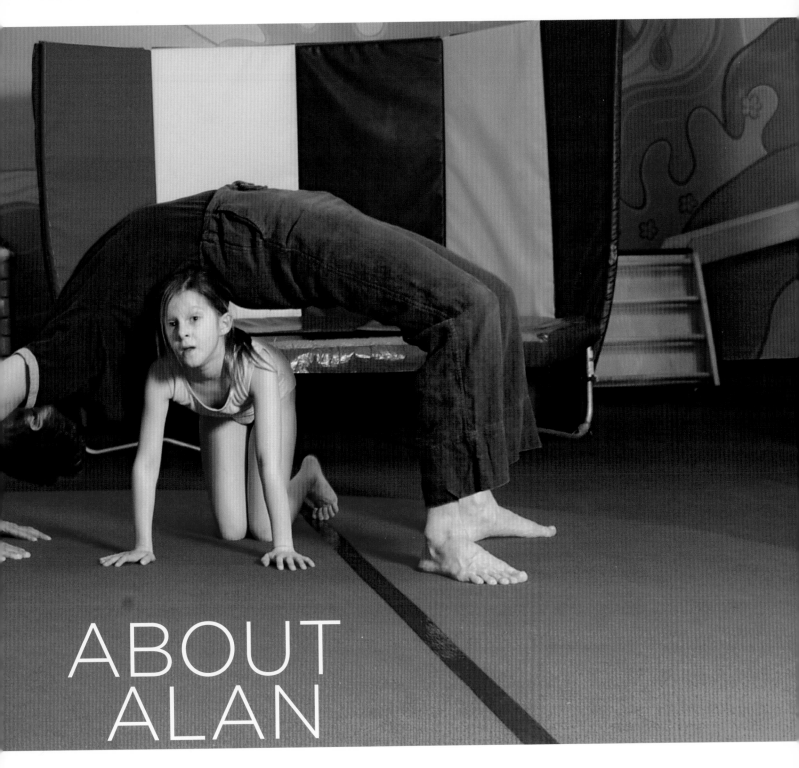

ABOUT ALAN

AGE	*40*
PROFESSION	*Project manager for an information technology firm*
TYPE OF PRACTICE	*Hatha Yoga*
LEVEL OF EXPERIENCE	*5 years*
MOST OBVIOUS BENEFIT OF THE PRACTICE TO ALAN	*Flexibility in body and mind, creative & playful connection with my daughters*
ALAN'S ADVICE TO OTHERS	*Practice the fundamentals regularly with purposeful attention so that when it's time to be spontaneous and playful you can trust your body to know its capabilities without having to think about it.*

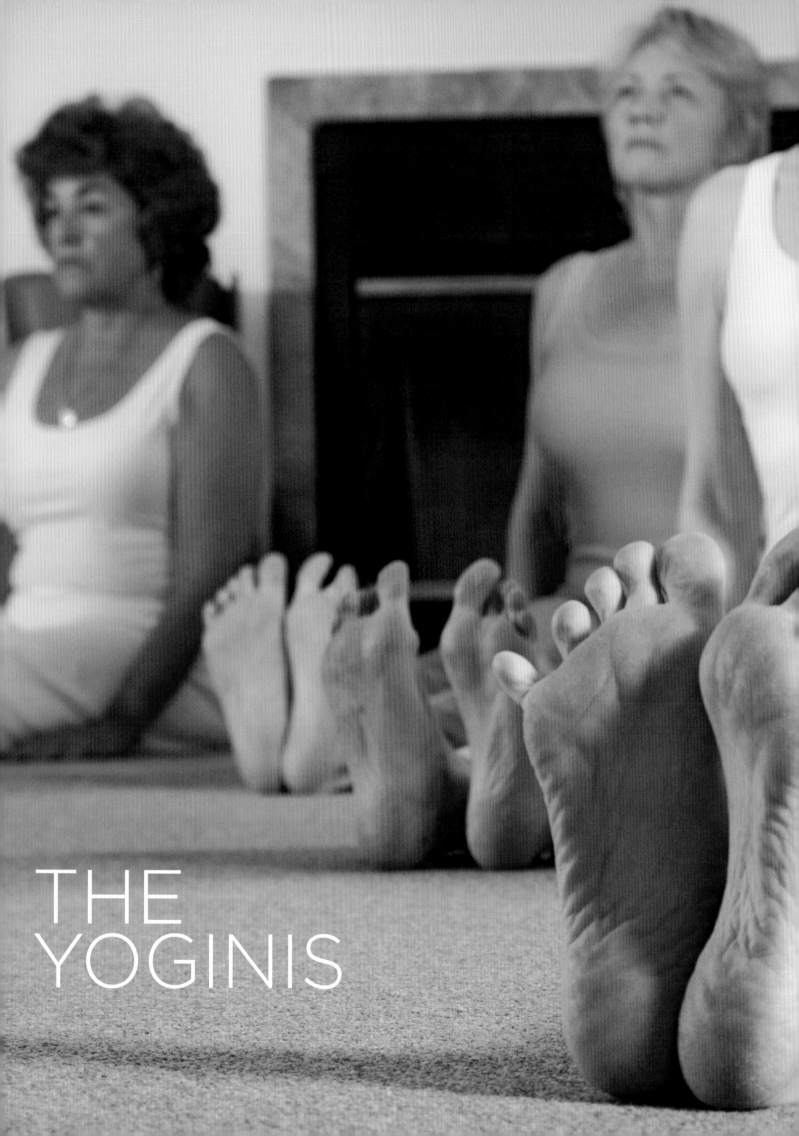

THE
YOGINIS

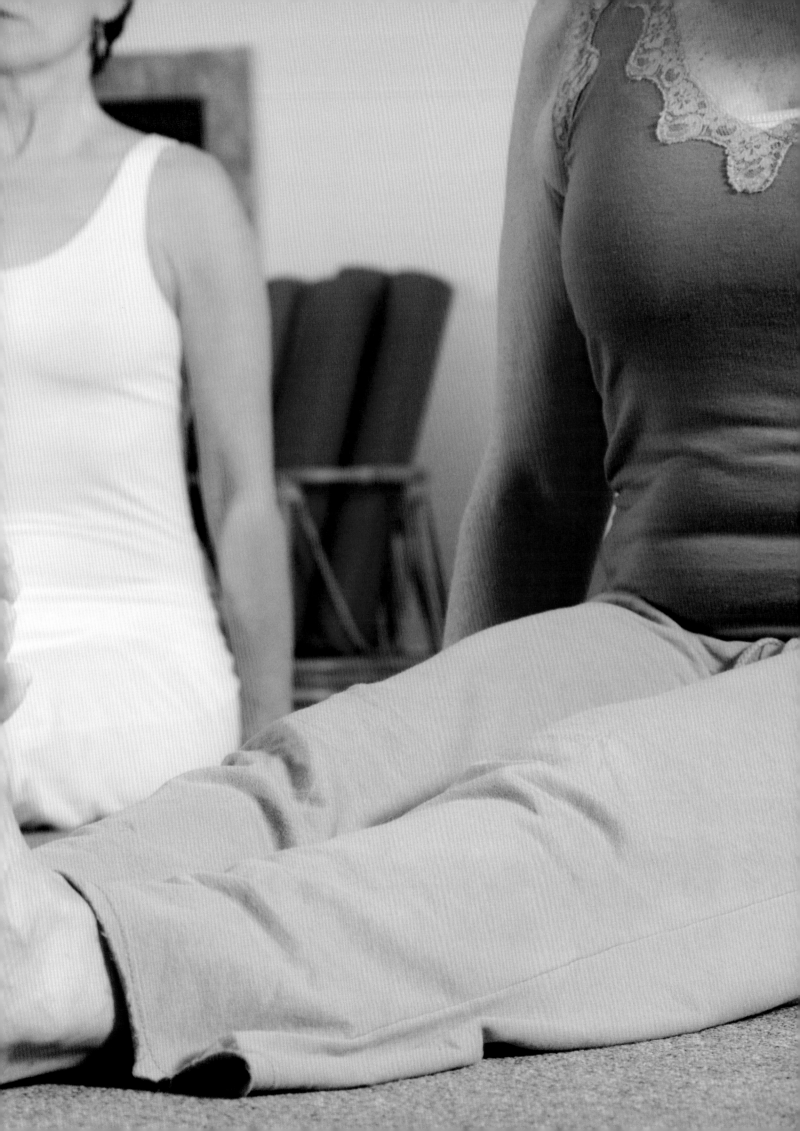

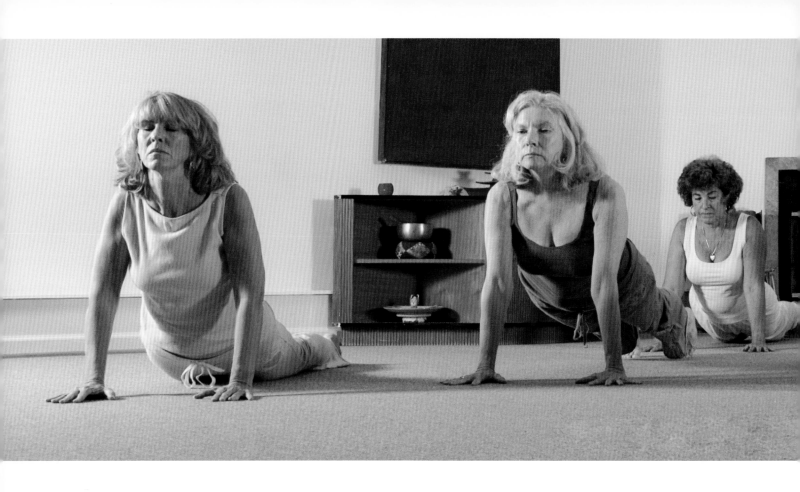

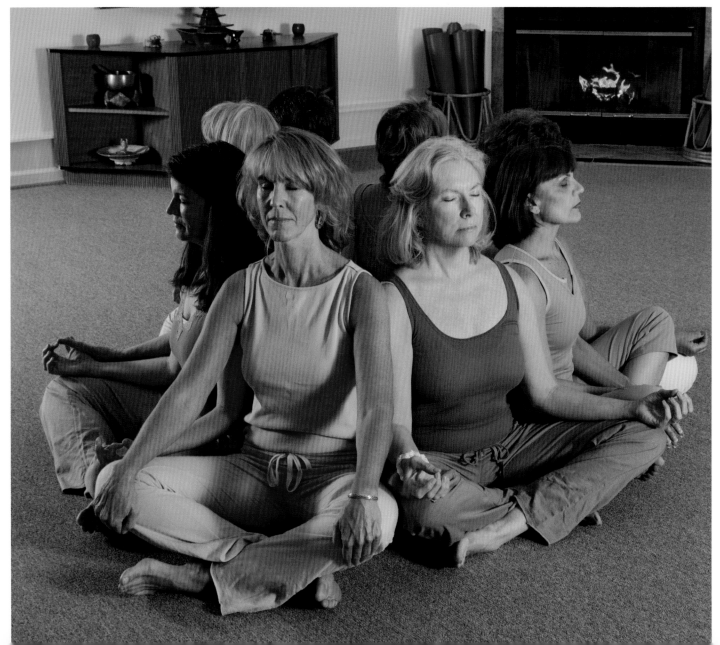

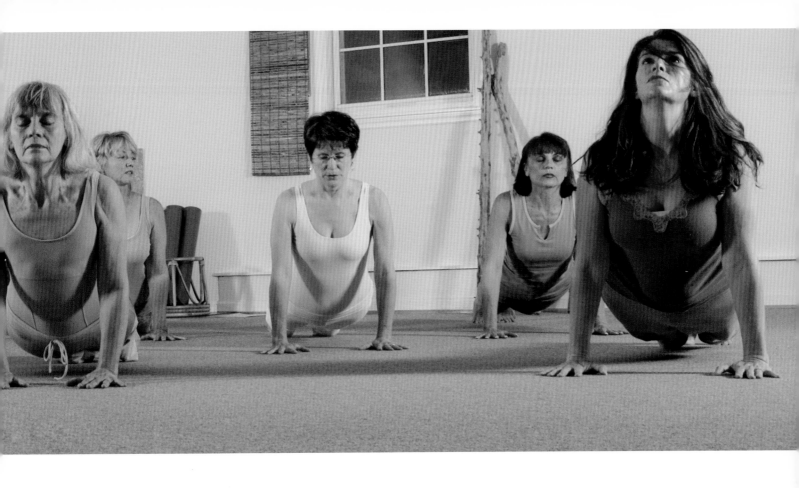

"We do not believe in ourselves until someone reveals that deep inside us something is valuable, worth listening to, worthy of our trust, sacred to our touch. Once we believe in ourselves we can risk curiosity, wonder, spontaneous delight or any experience that reveals the human spirit." E. E. CUMMINGS

EIGHT WOMEN, WITH BIRTHDATES SPANNING THREE DECADES, meet every Tuesday night for what all agree is a highlight of their week. They step into their shared sanctuary, checking their cares at the door. A chime sounds. A contented quiet fills the air. They roll yoga mats onto the floor in a sunburst pattern, circumscribing a sacred circle. They lower themselves to the floor, each in her own time. Legs cross, Lotus style. Gentle smiles make their way around the coterie, eyes meet softly and eight hearts beat as one.

Before they began taking yoga classes these women might have crossed paths unknowingly in the grocery store or at the movies, but the diversity of their careers and passions would have made it unlikely that they would become lifelong friends. What they did have in common was that they each felt drained, overtaxed and self-critical. From the full-time mom to the professional audiologist to the human resources expert and the elementary school principal, each maintained high-energy, demanding lives with little down time. Each came to yoga seeking relief from stress, hoping to achieve balance and serenity. What they happened upon exceeded their expectations.

It began with a closing ritual at the end of each class when their teacher would ask for questions or comments regarding the practice. At first, all the comments were cautiously polite and positive. Their teacher encouraged fearless honesty and little by little, they opened up, sharing frustrations, fears and personal foibles. Next came the birthday celebrations, which the yoginis describe as their "excuse for staying late to sip champagne and eat chocolates." As their interest in one another grew, they expanded their social

103

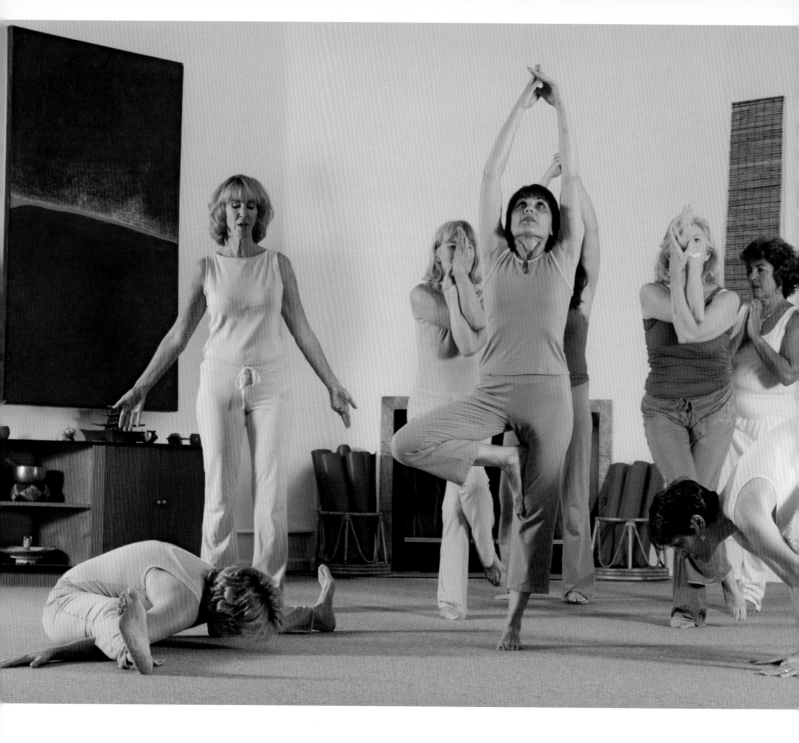

time to include book club meetings, movie and concert outings, and yoga retreats that featured spiritual explorations, poetry writing, and yoga in natural settings.

Together, the yoginis have explored their deepest feelings and grandest schemes. There is, by now, little they don't know about one another. "Without the yoga," says one, "I would never have found these kindred spirits." Another offers, "It's the greatest gift of my lifetime. I truly love these women and rely on them when all else seems lost." They have witnessed each other's achievements in yoga class, some pushing through fear while

practicing back-bends or handstands. Others are more challenged by "letting go" into the deep releases of forward folds or hip-openers. Whatever the challenge, they are steadfast supporters of each other, offering encouragement, humor and compassion.

When asked about the greatest value of their shared practice, the consensus is that yoga has helped them embrace the best and the worst that life has to offer, knowing that they have developed the strength and flexibility to move with agility through life, trusting that no matter what comes up, "We will never be alone."

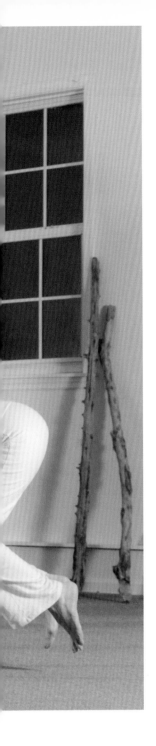

BETH	*Elementary school principal, age 49*
BIANCA	*Human resources specialist, age 54*
DEE	*Read about Dee on page 5*
JANE	*Audiologist, age 59*
JUDY	*Read about Judy on page 59*
KAREN	*Read about Karen on page 19*
MARVIS	*Read about Marvis on page 73*
MICHELE	*Full-time mother, age 43*
LEVEL OF EXPERIENCE	*Varied (more than 100 years, total)*
TYPE OF PRACTICE	*Hatha Yoga and related practices such as Martial Arts, Kundalini Yoga, Partner Yoga, Power Yoga, Restorative Practice, Meditation, and Celebration*
GREATEST BENEFIT OF THE PRACTICE TO THE YOGINIS	*Finding kindred spirits*
THE YOGINIS ADVICE TO OTHERS	*Find a yoga class and commit to it. Open your heart to everyone in the class, even those you can't relate to at first. Be honest and genuine when sharing your own insights. Forget about competition, embrace communion!*

ABOUT THE YOGINIS

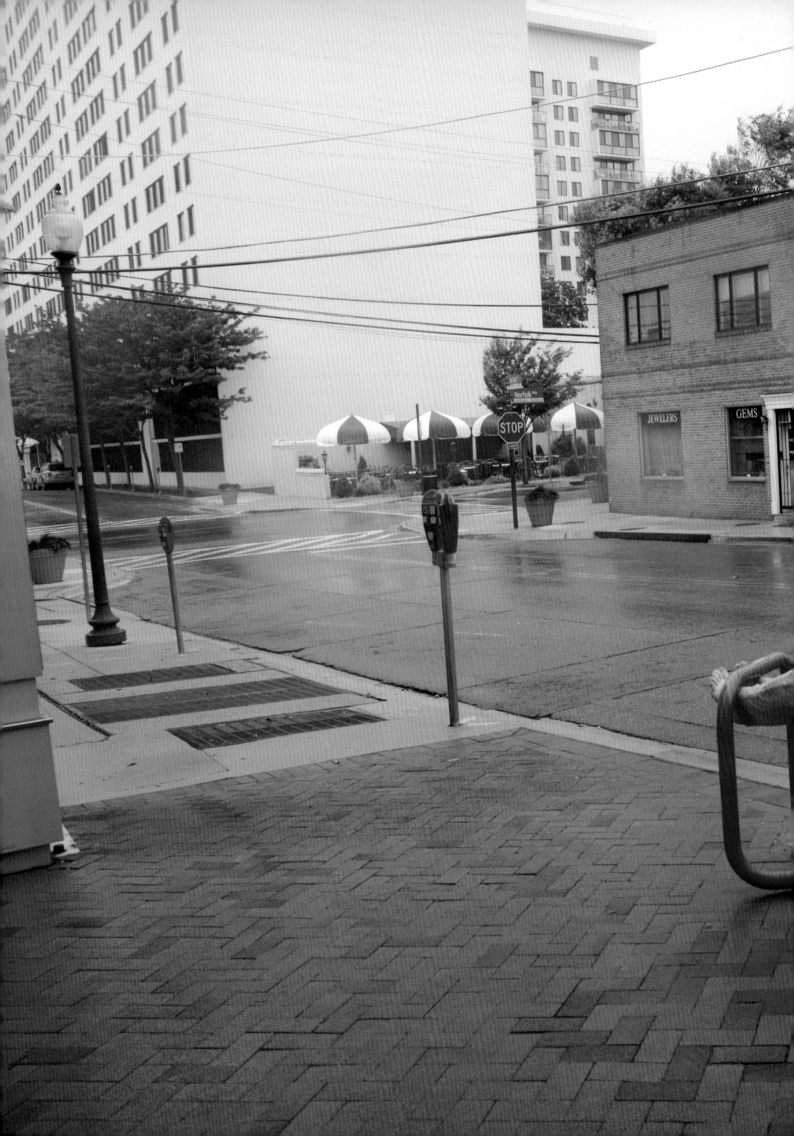

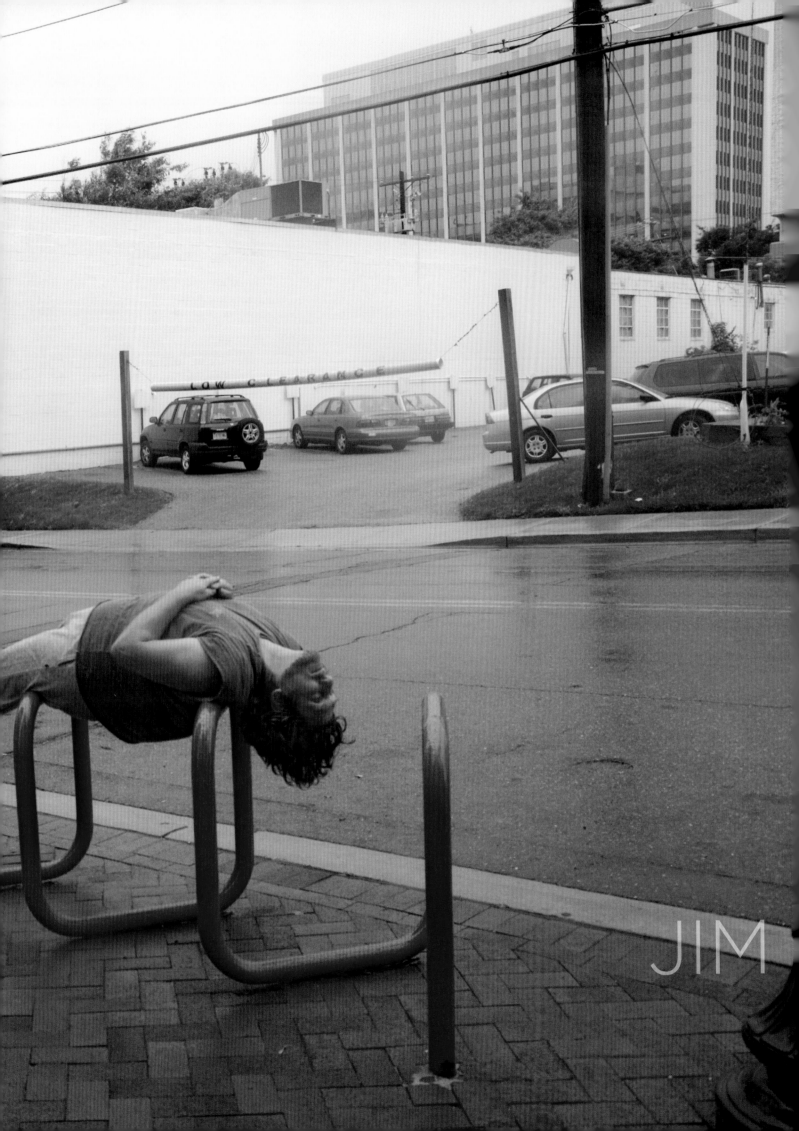

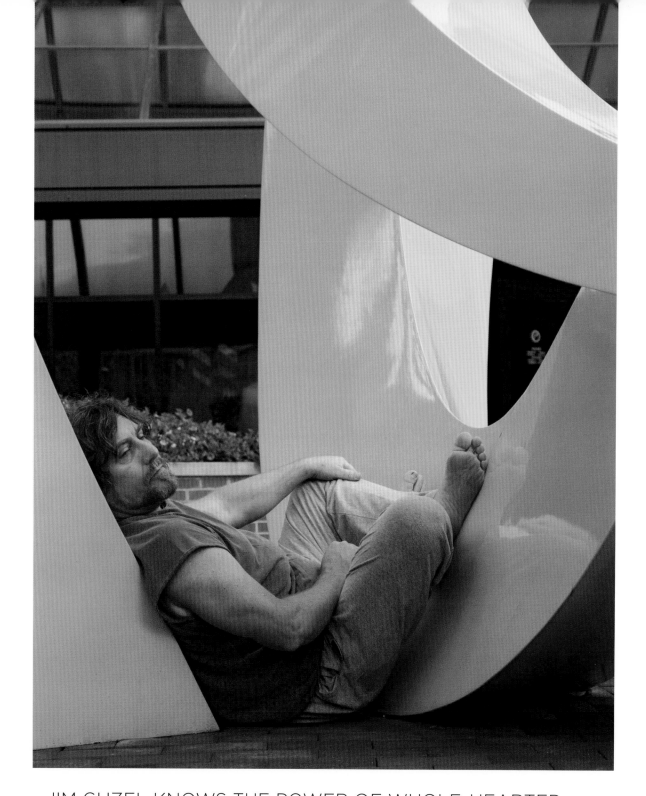

JIM GUZEL KNOWS THE POWER OF WHOLE-HEARTED INTERACTION WITH HIS ENVIRONMENT. While visiting his grandmother at age 9 or 10, Jim perused her yard, shaded by a variety of tall, stately trees, and resolved to climb every one. "There were dozens," he tells me, "and some had no low branches, making success improbable" for a young child. Undaunted, Jim tackled the challenge with a vigor that he continues to demonstrate as a professional photographer, 50 years later.

Jim has been a portrait photographer for 14 years and a gifted visual artist all his life. In elementary school in Pittsburgh, Jim was one of two students to be awarded a scholarship for a three year Saturday morning program to study art at the Carnegie Museum. In highly competitive art contests during high school, his artwork was awarded numerous accolades including a blue ribbon for his painting entitled "Veronica's Veil."

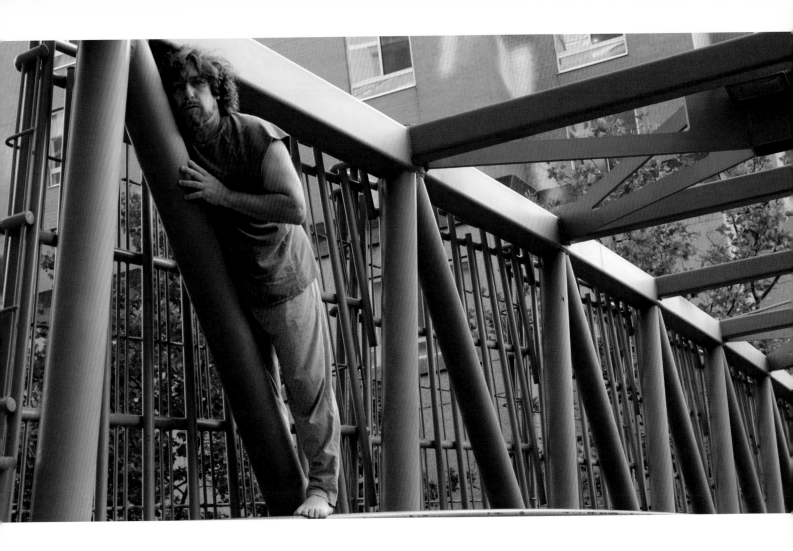

Jim was awarded a scholastic achievement scholarship and headed to Catholic University in Washington, D.C. to study architecture. But his youthful assuredness put him at odds with some faculty and in his pride Jim left the field, changing his major to Elementary Education. He graduated in 1972 with a Bachelor of Arts. He then went to work in the bustling restaurant industry of the nation's capital. For the next twenty-five years Jim's artistic flair would be primarily channeled into feeding and befriending the Washington power elite.

Jim never looked back. He worked hard and played hard. By the fall of 1994 he was in need of some R&R. He found himself drawn back to a stand of trees, this time in Shenandoah National Park. Fall foliage in the park is a must-see for D.C. locals and this had been a particularly stunning season. Jim brought a disposable camera

and spent the day hiking tough terrain and taking pictures. He was invigorated and eager to see the results. Jim was amazed when the prints came back (yes, these were the days of film developing.) "They were good," Jim says, eyes sparkling, "really good."

The artist in Jim sat up and took notice. The emboldened kid in him jumped for joy. No stranger to major life changes, Jim, now 45, shifted gears and threw himself into reverse to recapture his love of visual arts. Jim says, "The instant gratification of photography fit my personality." His love of people made portraiture an easy choice. Jim invested in a good camera and began photographing people in his spare time. After five years, Jim finally took the leap. Leaving the restaurant business, he established Aphrodite Photography, his portrait studio in Washington, D.C.

A natural athlete, Jim was drawn to

photographing people who loved to move their bodies. He teamed up with local choreographer, Tiffiny Wolins Gilreath, to create "Aspire," a unique approach to portrait photography in which Tiffiny would facilitate the client in originating "an improvised movement piece" fueled by unearthed emotion. The sessions gave rise to beautiful portraits but more important to Jim, the subjects reported that they were powerfully therapeutic, in some cases healing deeply rooted emotional trauma.

Jim's love of movement grew as he captured frame after frame of unfettered beauty in his clients. Tiffiny suggested that he, too, try creative movement as a tool for self-exploration and personal/professional growth. He was particularly drawn to the work of Gabrielle Roth and began attending 5Rhythms® workshops where he connected with others who loved to move. Jim grew more comfortable moving his body in spontaneous ways and his photography reflected increasing sensitivity and empathy with his subjects.

I met Jim during a dance workshop and we became fast friends. Our overlapping interests compelled us to work together and Jim agreed to photograph one of my yoga retreats. The topic of the retreat was one that resonated with Jim. "Oh, Beautiful!™" was designed to help women recognize and embrace their inherent beauty. Jim photographed the yoga sessions as creative art. He showed slides of the sessions at the end of each day. "The women got to see their own creativity which was more beautiful to them than any imitation of classic yoga poses," says Jim. "It was magical to see them acknowledge their own beauty."

Before that workshop, Jim, like most Westerners, had thought of yoga as an exercise regime. But again and again he witnessed participants releasing themselves from a shroud of negative self-assessment as they explored their natural beauty through creative and spontaneous yoga. He realized the parallel with his own work and came to see both as creating the "art of being you." He became even more excited to "help people see themselves as they are, not as they think they should be."

Equally excited by the outcome of the retreat, I approached Jim with an idea for a yoga book. It would not be a "how-to-do-yoga" book, but rather a "see how a creative yoga practice can enrich your life" book. Jim saw the book as an opportunity to "free people from self-imposed limitations by removing them from the typical reference points of yoga ... classic poses demonstrated by accomplished teachers and advanced practitioners." He happily signed on.

The project was underway! Models graciously volunteered. Each chose an environment or a concept that was emotionally important to them. "And in every case, fear came up," says Jim. "Every subject, no matter their level of expertise, had that moment of 'Is my yoga good enough to be photographed?' That's when our jobs really started." Jim approached every session with the absolute unyielding belief that it would work. His confidence was infectious. "The subject has to forget about doing yoga," Jim says, "they have to just trust their bodies. Then, everything gets to flow without the inner critic getting in the way."

When Jim was asked whether his participation in the book inspired him to practice yoga he chuckled and said, "Actually, no." But, he recalled the climbing, twisting, balancing, and bending it took to do the shoots and added, "I guess I was doing a sort of photography yoga the entire time."

So, what better way to enrich Jim's life as a creative artist than to take him out from behind the camera and have him play in an environment of his choosing? Jim accepted the challenge and decided

110

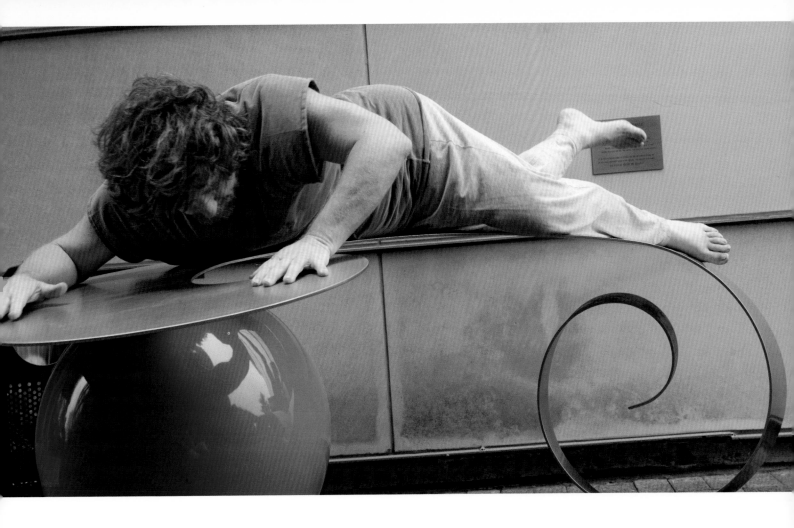

to try a creative yoga practice in an urban environment. "As a student of architecture and a visual artist, I thought it would be appropriate," says Jim. So, witness here the "coming full circle" of the determined kid, the bold student, playful dancer and award-winning visual artist.

Jim and I reversed roles. I took the camera and he took to the task of creating his yoga. (We both gained a greater appreciation for the other's skill.) Afterward, he had to admit, "Adding creativity to your yoga brings enrichment to your everyday life. The mundane becomes the beautiful."

Jim's hope in participating in this book is that every reader stretches beyond the ordinary in their lives to experience the joy and beauty of the creative process. Jim concludes, "Everyone should know himself or herself as a creative artist. Doing creative yoga is a terrific path to that end."

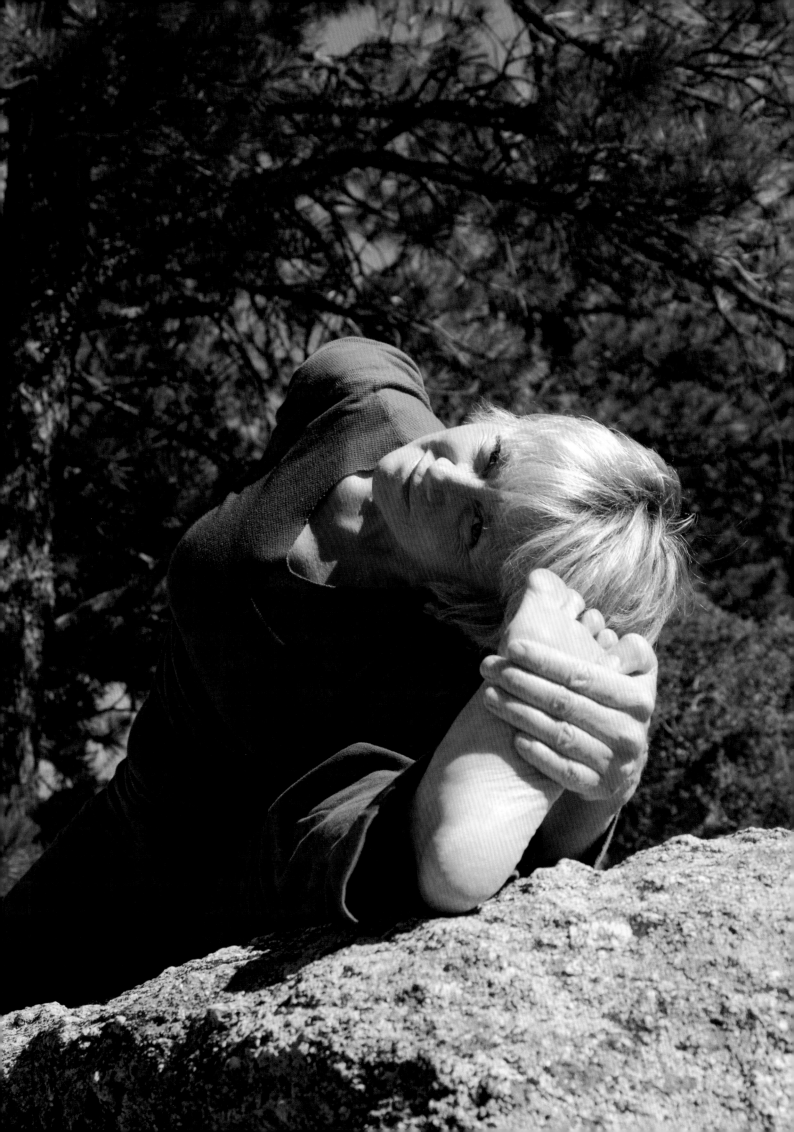

I WAS BORN A YOGI ... AND SO WERE YOU, though most of us need help to remember when mind and body were one. The experience faded as we grew.

My earliest memory is of peering through the wooden bars of my crib. I couldn't have been more than two years old. I wanted to explore ... and I did. My gaze transported me through the bedroom window and beyond the tiny enclosure of our back yard. It seemed to me that I hovered above a far off field of golden weeds. I can still feel the swaying of those sunlit stalks in my body. I can still align my breath with the rhythm of the breeze. I can still feel the freedom of physical and mental release, in sharp contrast to the unwelcome confinement of my prescribed naptime.

I was the type of child who could not stay still. I explored everything with my body, just like children the world over. I put things in my mouth. I wriggled around in dirt. I climbed trees and hung upside-down from branches. Once, around the age of seven, I scrambled to a neighbor's rooftop, causing my mother (and our neighbor) great distress.

My parents were of a generation whose primary rule was, "Children should be seen and not heard." My constant questioning about how things worked must have been an annoyance. I remember, around the age of eight, asking my exasperated mother, "Why does the moon follow us when we drive?" She sighed and stated flatly, "To make you ask questions." For some reason, her response that day was the one that finally silenced me. I stopped asking questions out loud. Instead, I honed the sharpest implement of understanding available to me, my body.

I became a stealth learner. I silently practiced being a squirrel, a bird, a pony. I tried to absorb, through my skin, the smell of grass and the feel of water. I imagined that I could store these sensations deep in my bones and revisit them at will. I learned about people, too, by putting myself "in their skin." (Today, this skill known as "kinesthetic empathy," is taught to body psychotherapists as a tool for diagnosis and treatment.)

By the time I was ten or eleven years old, I had developed quite a talent for molding and moving my body in ways that mimicked my surroundings. I was convinced that I knew exactly how it felt to be a tree, a rock, a worm, a brook. I had taken ballet lessons since the age of four and hypothesized that the muscular control necessary to perform pliés and jetés was enhancing my abilities to know the world around me. So, I practiced with greater intensity.

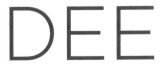

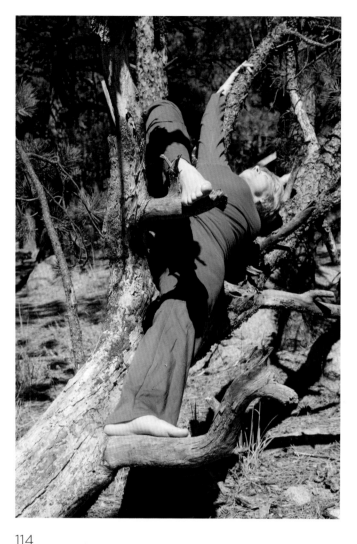

It occurred to me that the very act of breathing required a miraculous orchestration of body parts, many of which were invisible to the eye but could be felt and imagined. My attention turned to subtler levels of muscle control. It must have been strange for my parents to witness the determined inward focus of my mind as I sat for hours, literally navel gazing —watching my belly rise and fall with each inhale and exhale. I thrilled at the discovery that I could be in constant motion while appearing to be still. I would rediscover this delight later in life through the practice of hatha yoga, in which postures are held for minutes at a time while breath moves freely to bring vitality to each pose.

Maybe it was the inward focus. Maybe it was the stillness of mind. Maybe it was an accident, but one day while intentionally rolling the muscles of my belly, I "heard" a phrase arise from deep within. "My body is my temple," it said. Like a carillon, a harmony rang through my bones and I knew the truth. "My body is my temple."

My family wasn't particularly religious. Our attendance at the nearby Presbyterian Church was irregular. When we did go, I enjoyed sitting in the balcony and visualized myself leaping, monkey-like, from railing to chandelier. I could feel, in my body, the joy and excitement of swinging over the head of our stern minister and the colorful hats of the parishioners who sat before him, some rapt in reverence, some nodding off. It was then that I realized the power of imagination. I could capture the thrill of swinging through a jungle canopy even while sitting quietly in church.

"My body is my temple." I heard it over and over in my mind, like a favorite song. "My body is my church," I explained to my mother, insisting that I no longer needed to be a part of a congregation. Puzzled

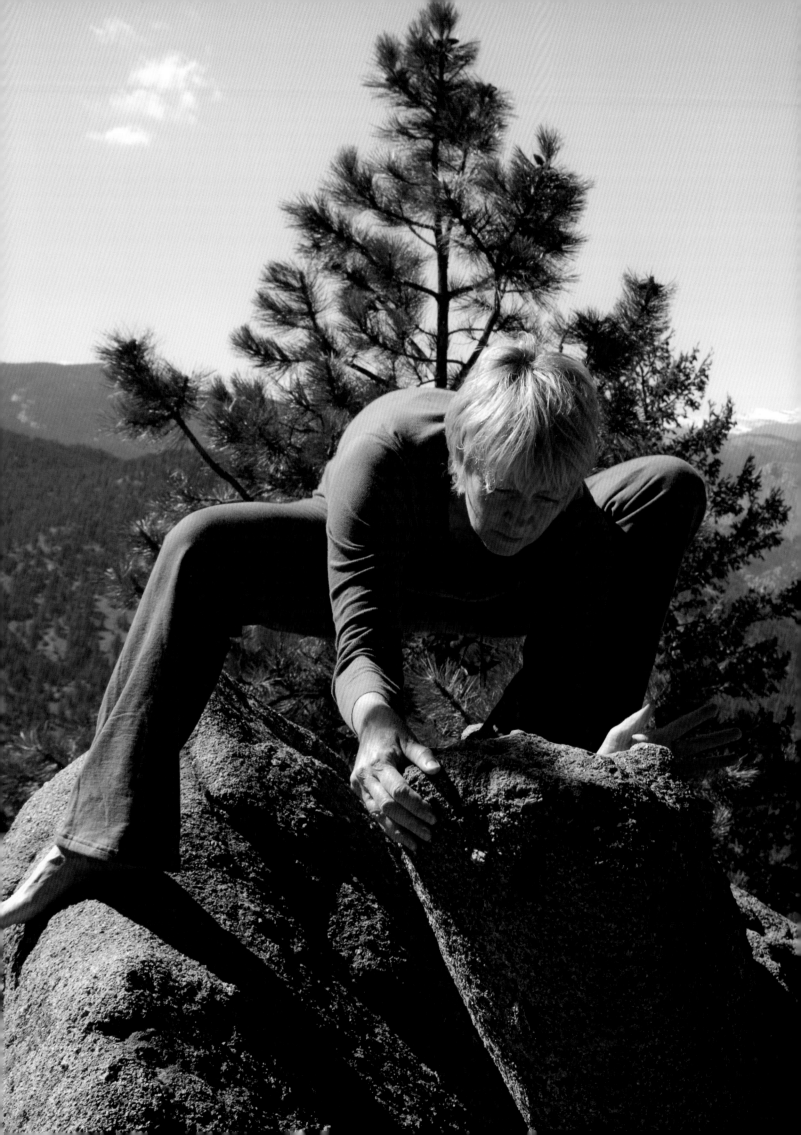

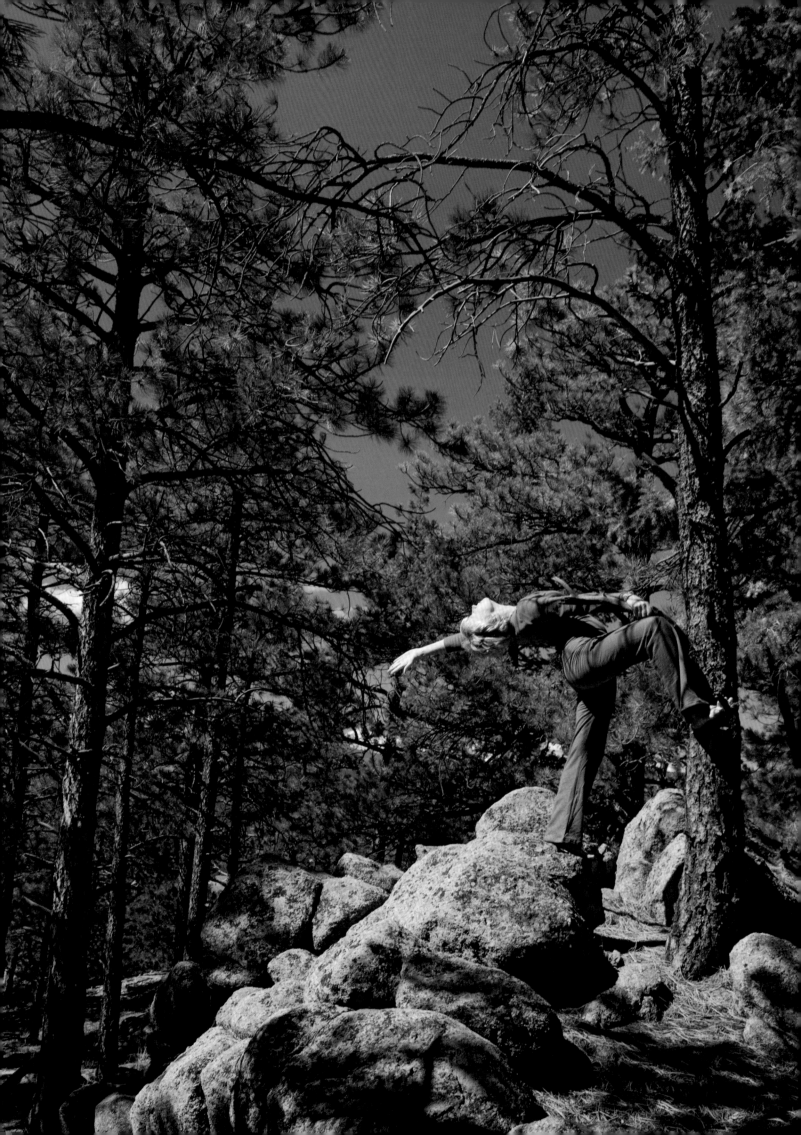

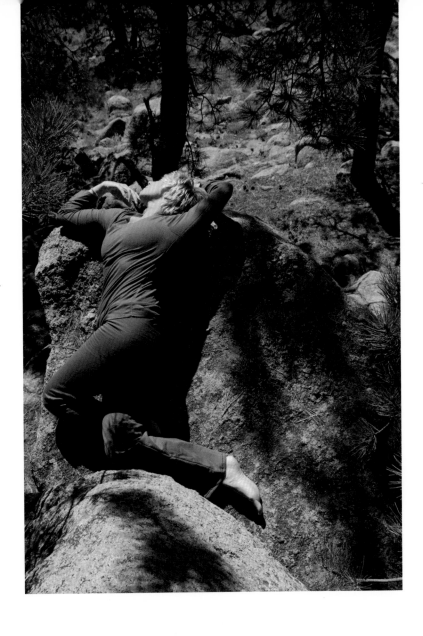

and exhausted, she stared at me silently. I think she may have been relieved, for never again did she insist on squeezing me into my Sunday best. My body was my temple and, to me, that meant keeping it unencumbered ... no more scratchy crinolines or pointy-toed patent leather shoes. My Sunday mornings were spent barefoot in a nearby stream or perched in the crook of a friendly oak tree.

The reverence I felt became a spiritual template for the rest of my life. To this day, when I practice yoga, I allow myself to embody the mountain, the tree, the cobra, the cat and the cow. Every yoga pose has an essence which is typically expressed in the name of the pose and can be experienced in the body and mind. The essence of Camel, for example, can be felt in the upward curve of the front body as arms and head drape back toward feet.

The uplifted tail of Downward-Facing Dog emulates the canine invitation to play. The arch of the torso in Crescent Moon perfectly conveys that lunar phase.

The beauty of yoga, as I see it, is that it provides a foundation for self-awareness and spiritual development. The classic poses or asanas offer a blueprint for how to build a strong body and supple mind that ultimately becomes the "temple" for a life of reverence and awe. From the smallest particle of dust to the furthest reaches of the cosmos, Creation holds vast mysteries. Yoga is at once the microscope and the telescope. Whether looking deeply within or expanding into boundlessness, the art and science of yoga offers clarity of vision and purpose.

My vision is a world in which peace and harmony prevail, a world that cultivates compassion and acceptance, and values

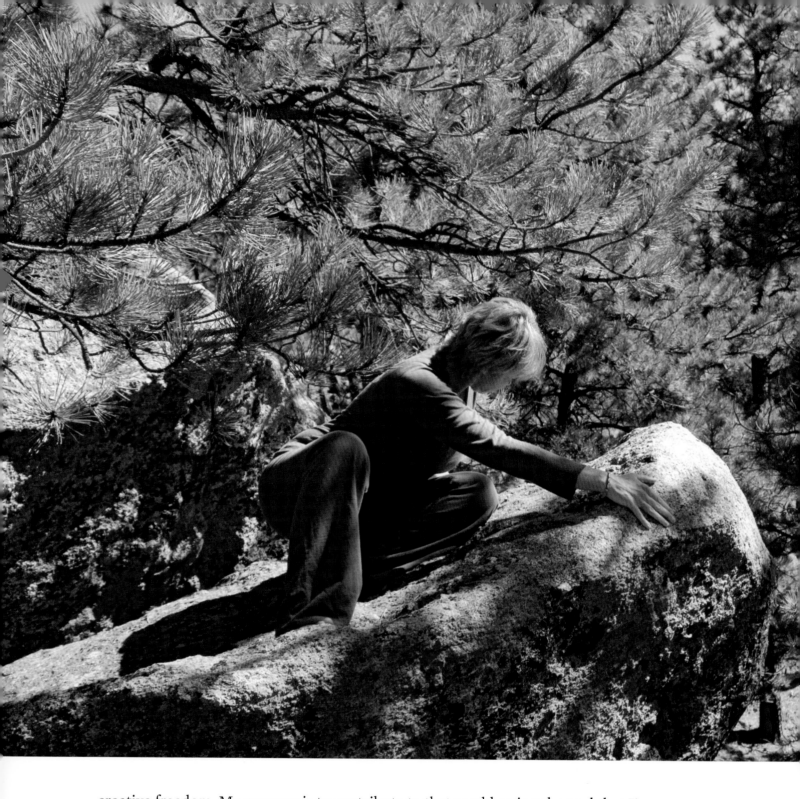

creative freedom. My purpose is to contribute to that world, using the tool that I've sharpened throughout my lifetime, my kinesthetic sense. By uniting with nature and humankind through yoga, I have reached my personal goal of balance, harmony and freedom of expression. Through my teachings I have encouraged many others, like the subjects in this book, to do the same. This book is an offering and an invitation to all who read it to stretch beyond the confines of your physical and mental habits. Break free of your intellectual conditioning and risk feeling the fool for the higher purpose of coming to know yourself. You are a divine creation. Your existence is a golden braid of body, mind, and spirit woven into the fabric of the Great Mystery.

Yoga means union. Step onto a yoga mat with an intention to unite mind and body. Spirit will arise. Step off your mat and bring your spirit creatively into the world. You will come to know your place in the cosmos. You will begin to understand, deep

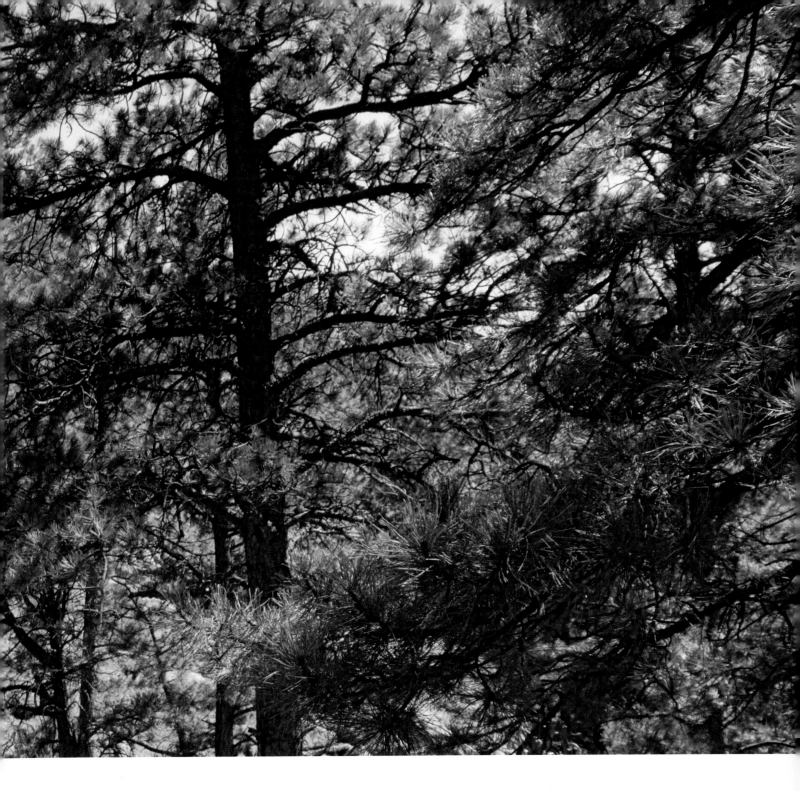

within your bones that you are one with all that is. You will no longer look into the eyes of another without seeing a reflection of yourself. You will no longer feel separate from the air you breathe or the ground on which you walk. You will know every expression of life. And you will be free.

~Namaste~

"The divine light in me recognizes the divine light in you. When you do the same in return, we are one."